PENGUIN BOOKS

changing *shape*

Kathryn Bramwell is the managing director of Changing Shape, which runs exercise classes for pregnant women and new mothers. She graduated as a physiotherapist in 1978, then worked in country Victoria and community health centres, and qualified as an exercise-to-music leader with VicFit in 1983. Her special area of interest is women's health and she has conducted specialised exercise classes and health programs for pregnant women and new mothers since 1984, when she founded Changing Shape as a single weekly exercise class to help herself get fit after the birth of her second child. She is a past president of the Women's Health Physiotherapy Group (Victorian Chapter) of the Australian Physiotherapy Association. She regularly lectures on pregnancy exercise to both the general public and the fitness industry.

Margaret Sherburn graduated as a physiotherapist in 1970, and in 1989 qualified as an exercise-to-music leader with VicFit. She has worked in Victoria and overseas. From 1986 to 1994 she worked with Changing Shape, initially as an exercise leader and later as a director. She regularly lectures to physiotherapy students and the fitness industry on the relationship of anatomy and kinesiology to exercise prescription. She is presently tutoring at the School of Physiotherapy, Faculty of Medicine, Dentistry and Health Sciences, University of Melbourne, and conducts childbirth preparation programs at South Eastern Private Hospital.

Both Kathryn and Margaret have personal experience of pregnancy, childbirth and motherhood. Each has a 13-year-old daughter and an 11-year-old son.

changing *shape*

Exercising for Fitness and Wellbeing During and After Pregnancy

KATHRYN BRAMWELL AND MARGARET SHERBURN

PENGUIN BOOKS

The two exercise programs in this book have been designed for readers to do at home. While every care has been taken in researching and compiling the information in this book, it is in no way intended to replace or supersede professional medical advice. Neither the authors nor the publisher may be held responsible for any action or claim resulting from the use of this book or any information contained in it.

PENGUIN BOOKS

Published by the Penguin Group
Penguin Books Ltd, 27 Wrights Lane,
London W8 5TZ, England
Penguin Books USA Inc., 375 Hudson Street,
New York, New York 10014, USA
Penguin Books Australia Ltd, Ringwood,
Victoria, Australia
Penguin Books Canada Ltd, 10 Alcorn Avenue,
Toronto, Ontario, Canada M4V 3B2
Penguin Books (NZ) Ltd, 182-190 Wairau Road,
Auckland 10, New Zealand

Penguin Books Ltd, Registered Offices:
Harmondsworth, Middlesex, England

First published in Australia by Viking 1995
Published in Penguin Books 1995
10 9 8 7 6 5 4 3 2 1

Copyright © Changing Shape Pty Ltd, 1995
All rights reserved

The moral right of the author has been asserted

Typeset in Sabon
Photography by Sally-Ann Balharrie
Printed in Australia by Australian Print Group,
Maryborough, Victoria, Australia

contents

Foreword *vii*
Acknowledgements *viii*
Introduction *ix*

PART ONE
FITNESS AND PREGNANCY

1 BECOMING FIT   2

Preparing your body *3*
How will exercise help? *5*

2 HOW YOUR BODY CHANGES
   DURING PREGNANCY   7

The hidden changes *8*
Pelvic-floor bracing *16*
The obvious changes *17*
Abdominal bracing: 'press-studs', waistline
    gathering and pelvic tucks *22*

3 GUIDELINES FOR MINIMISING RISKS   24

Seeking advice *25*
Your and your baby's health *25*
Your previous experience of exercise *26*
Risky exercise choices *28*
Warning signs *29*
Pregnancy exercise guidelines *34*

4 DESIGNING A SAFE EXERCISE PROGRAM   36

Controlling weight gain *36*
Preparing for childbirth *37*
Maintaining fitness *38*
Components of a fitness plan *38*
What type of exercise is best? *42*

5 CHOOSING THE RIGHT AEROBIC EXERCISE *48*

Walking *49*
Swimming *51*
Stationary bike riding *52*
Low-impact aerobics *53*
Gym program *54*
Step, slide, circuit and box-a-cise classes *55*

PART TWO
HOME EXERCISE PROGRAM FOR PREGNANCY

6 BEGINNING THE EXERCISES *60*

Following the home exercise program *61*

THE PROGRAM *64*

PART THREE
HOME EXERCISE PROGRAM FOR
AFTER CHILDBIRTH

7 GETTING YOUR BODY BACK INTO SHAPE *104*

When can you start exercising? *105*
What changes happen after childbirth? *106*
Following the home exercise program *109*

THE PROGRAM *112*

changing *shape*

ACKNOWLEDGEMENTS

We would like to thank in particular: Caroline Pizzey of Penguin Books with whom the original idea for this book was conceived; Dr Robin Bell, Dr Kate Duncan and Robyn Compton for their help with editing the copy and for adding their expertise in the respective fields of pregnancy exercise, obstetrics and gynaecology, and dietetics; Elke Lushington and baby Kathleen, and Nicole Brown and baby Ashley, for their patience and enthusiasm during the photographic sessions, and also the other Changing Shape clients who were involved in the class photographic session; and the Yarrbat Sports and Fitness Centre, Melbourne, their wonderful staff (especially Paul, Marley and Tiffany) and their members for their help with the gym photographs.

We would also like to thank the present and previous staff and the many clients who have participated in the Changing Shape program since our early days in 1984. It is our constant reliance on their real life experience that makes the Changing Shape exercise program so relevant to pregnant women and new mothers today.

introduction

Changing Shape has been written for pregnant women and new mothers who wish to gain or maintain general fitness. It is also a guide for women wishing to prepare physically and actively for childbirth and recovery after the birth (whether vaginal or caesarean). For women who are competent athletes or sportswomen, the book will serve as a reminder that all pregnant women experience the physical, physiological and psychological changes of pregnancy and that they therefore need to discuss their training regime with an exercise consultant.

The exercises offered in *Changing Shape* are the result of our years of experience running the Changing Shape exercise classes. When Changing Shape was established in 1984, aerobics had just begun to create a storm in the fitness world, but there was very little information available about what exercise was safe for pregnant women and new mothers. In *Changing Shape*, we have combined our physiotherapists' understanding of exercise physiology and exercise prescription with our knowledge gained from leading the Changing Shape exercise program, and drawn on current research in the field, to provide safe exercise alternatives for healthy pregnant women and new mothers.

The book is divided into three parts. Part 1 provides information and advice on exercising during pregnancy. Part 2 offers a

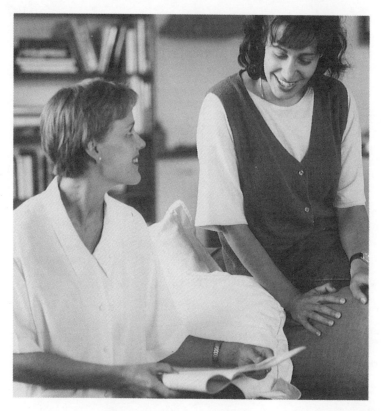

Home Exercise Program for Pregnancy, which gives specific exercises for strength and flexibility, arranged so that users work logically from one position to the next. Just the exercise names and photos will be enough to remind readers of the exercises after they have done the program a few times. Part 3 covers the transition to motherhood and offers a Home Exercise Program for After Childbirth, which can include the baby. Parts 2 and 3 also give women specific tips on how to vary the exercises, firstly as their pregnancies progress and secondly as they become stronger after the birth.

It is presumed that all women will be thoroughly screened by their medical consultant before they undertake the exercises in this book. For most women this will be enough. (Medical consultant is the term used throughout to describe the qualified medical practitioner who has the responsibility of monitoring the pregnancy, such as an obstetrician, doctor or midwife.)

Advice from an exercise consultant will enhance your individual programming, but in most cases is not essential before you undertake the home exercise programs given in the book. Exercise consultants should have a thorough understanding of exercise and the implications of pregnancy. Specialist pregnancy exercise consultants are available in some communities; they have a health or physical science background (they are graduates in, for example, physiotherapy, exercise physiology or human movement), plus a specialist qualification or experience in the field of exercise during pregnancy.

The focus of *Changing Shape* is on safe exercise at home and the benefits of exercise for both mother and baby. Exercise is a great way to prepare the body for the tasks of mothering.

After all, taking care of your baby could be said to begin with taking care of yourself!

fitness and pregnancy

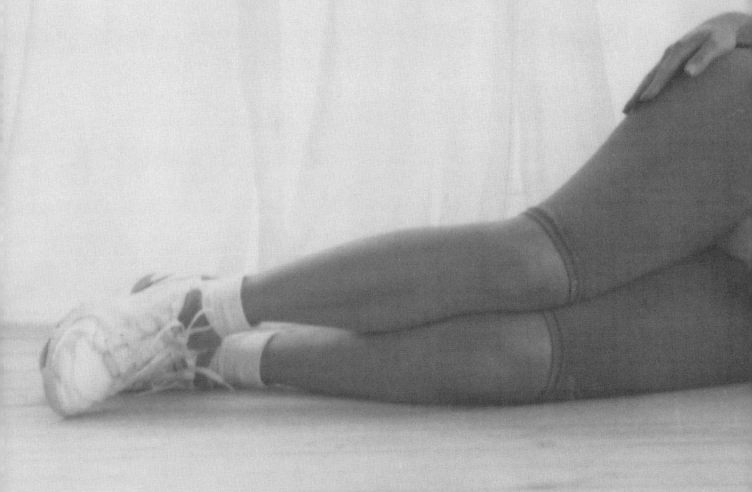

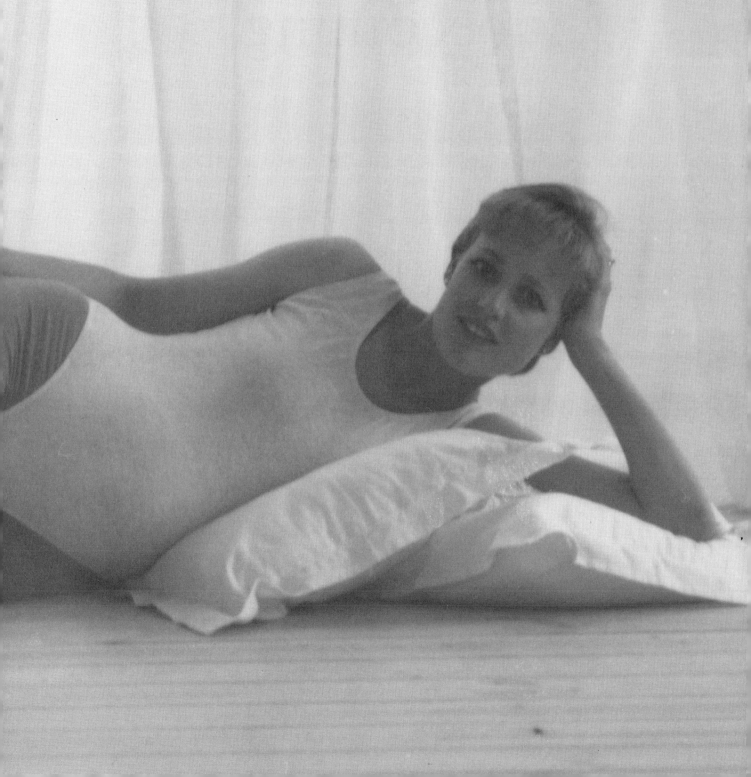

p a r t   o n e

becoming fit

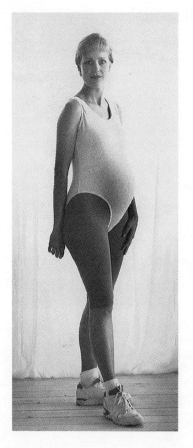

Except in the world of cartoons where a stork appears on the doorstep with your baby, motherhood is not achieved by magic. In the real world, becoming a mother involves the four stages of becoming pregnant, being pregnant, giving birth and caring for your new baby. Once you have conceived, you can't leave the pregnancy behind in the office or deal with it tomorrow. Your body is directly involved in the process twenty-four hours a day.

It sometimes helps to consider becoming a mother in the same way as you would approach beginning a new career. Each stage will require preparation, mastering new skills and adjusting to changes before you begin to feel competent. And, of course, with this career there is also the excitement and challenge of growing and nurturing a new life.

Many women today feel they have to be superwomen: that they have to add pregnancy and motherhood to their existing workload without relinquishing any part of it or adding any assistance. You may be lucky and cope with the increased load, but it is far better to plan so that you have as smooth a transition to motherhood as possible. To achieve a successful balance in your life, ask your self the following questions.

1   What is best for my baby?
2   What is best for me?
3   What is best for my family?

The priority of these questions may change, but each decision you make will have an impact on all your family. Your decisions also may be different from those of others; however, your aim should always be to keep everything in balance to achieve the best experience, given your personal circumstances.

Caring for the baby begins with the mother. It is widely accepted that the health of both the woman and her pregnancy influences the outcome of pregnancy. So, when planning to become pregnant, you should also plan to make healthy lifestyle choices. They will help you to cope physically with the changes of pregnancy and should provide the best environment for your baby's growth and development. The choices you make with regard to nutrition, smoking, drugs, exercise and rest will influence not only your health but your baby's as well.

The physical condition of your body is very important for both your energy and your comfort during pregnancy and for your ability to look after your newborn baby. Recent research on exercise during pregnancy supports the view that there are positive health benefits associated with exercising regularly throughout pregnancy and returning to exercise shortly after your baby is born.

PREPARING YOUR BODY

As an expectant mother in today's world, you will probably need to introduce or maintain regular exercise in your daily routine to prepare yourself physically for childbirth and motherhood. In previous generations women were responsible for the house and they automatically exercised as they knelt and squatted doing their housework. They also had little choice but to walk everywhere. Now we get in the car to go even short distances; to

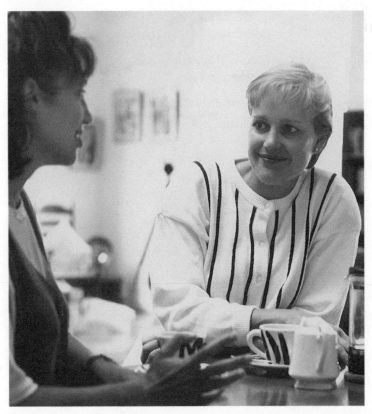

Talking with a friend who has had a baby lets you share your experiences.

heat our houses we flick a switch rather than chop or collect wood; and we have replaced scrubbing floors with vacuuming!

All women today will benefit from being generally fit; that is, from having stamina, strength and flexibility. However, pregnant women need to be encouraged to become specifically fit for pregnancy, childbirth and motherhood. Obviously, the type of exercise program they participate in will vary according to their health, lifestyle and previous exercise experience. Nevertheless, whatever the previous experience or level of fitness, there are essential exercises that should be added to every pregnant woman's program.

A well-balanced exercise program for pregnancy should include:

- a warm-up to prepare your body for activity
- aerobic-fitness activities, such as walking or swimming, at levels that are appropriate for your developing baby
- strengthening exercises that target the muscle groups most stressed by pregnancy
- body awareness exercises to help you manage your changing posture
- flexibility exercises for your lower back, pelvis and hips
- squatting and pelvic rocking in preparation for childbirth
- a cool-down to prevent injury.

The exercises in the Home Exercise Program for Pregnancy given in Part 2 will provide you with a balanced complement to the selection of aerobic activities outlined in Chapter 5.

Coping with your changing shape

Some women will embrace their change of shape as an expression of full womanhood. Other women, however, will find the inevitable changes in body shape associated with becoming a mother difficult to reconcile with their body image of themselves. Many women are used to being valued for their appearance. Fashion dictates the norm, and today that norm is decidedly slim. The pregnant shape may be natural but only a small percentage of women in our community are pregnant at any one time, so on many occasions pregnant women may feel the 'odd one out'.

Unfortunately, the pregnant shape is often confused with fatness and in our present society not many women aspire to look fat! Yet physiologically it is important that you, as well as your developing baby, gain weight in pregnancy. It is normal for this weight to accumulate around the hips, thighs, bottom and breasts. It is also normal for some to remain when you are breastfeeding.

The patterns of weight gain vary from woman to woman and from pregnancy to pregnancy. Some women gain less weight than recommended, have large babies and successfully breastfeed. Others gain more than recommended, gain it early, and yet still return to their normal weight after the birth. You need to discuss any concerns about weight gain throughout your pregnancy with your medical consultant or a dietician.

Your shape will be ever changing in pregnancy. It is to a large extent independent of your actions, although how you manage your energy input (food) and energy output (activity level) can alter the extent of the change, and hence your reaction to it. However, pregnancy is not the time to use exercise as a means of reducing your essential weight gain, but rather as a time for you to use exercise, in association with healthy eating, to limit unnecessary weight gain.

HOW WILL EXERCISE HELP?

The changes in your body during pregnancy usually reflect the development of your baby. How your body reacts is individual and can be affected by your fitness level. In general, exercising regularly will probably help you cope with the changes that are occurring in your body because you will feel you are contributing positively to your health and doing something normal. However, the changes in your body mean that your exercise choices should be different from those made when you were not pregnant.

There are now two of you exercising together, you and your baby.

Working out in a specialised pregnancy exercise class with other pregnant women will help you acknowledge the presence of your baby and accept your changing shape as normal and desirable. However, as this book shows, you can also successfully exercise at home.

There are various types of exercise suitable for pregnancy that focus on the exercise goals of aerobic fitness, strength and flexibility. Aerobic exercise, such as walking, swimming and cycling, involves using large-muscle groups to improve your cardiovascular and respiratory fitness. Some of the benefits of aerobic exercise during pregnancy are feeling physically capable of continuing your normal activities for longer into your pregnancy and having more energy in reserve to enjoy the pleasures of life and motherhood. Strengthening the specific postural muscles affected by the changes of pregnancy will improve your muscle tone, and lessen any backache and pelvic-joint discomfort. Improving your flexibility may help lessen the physical discomforts of pregnancy and specifically prepare your body for labour.

Other benefits reported by women who exercise regularly in specially designed programs for pregnancy are:

▶ a feeling of wellbeing
▶ easier management of weight gain during pregnancy
▶ less tiredness at the end of the day and better sleep at night
▶ a sense of poise and grace of movement
▶ confidence and trust in their body's ability to give birth.

An exercise program that emphasises all components of fitness is ideal for you in pregnancy. Your general health, the health of your pregnancy and your previous exercise experience will influence where you start and how much you do. The changes in your body may mean that your exercise choices will be different from those available to you when you were not pregnant. Obviously there will be differences between what is suitable for an athlete and what someone just starting out can cope with. The information in the following chapters will help you to develop an exercise program that is suitable for you and your baby.

Note Before you start any exercise program during pregnancy you should discuss your plans with your medical consultant.

how your body changes during pregnancy

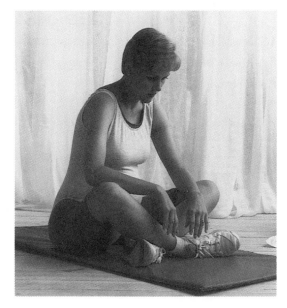

As your baby grows inside you, you will become aware of obvious changes in your body's shape. Less obviously, there are internal physiological changes occurring also, which are essential for your baby's growth and development. While the extent of both these obvious and hidden changes may differ, they all occur in all women.

What are the changes happening within your body? The hidden ones are the physiological changes needed to provide the right environment for your baby's development. Changes such as heart enlargement and increased blood volume are not visible, but they are very important factors to consider when planning your exercise program. The obvious changes are – well, obvious! Your weight gain and your altered posture are very visible and can't be ignored.

How will the changes affect your choice of exercise? All of them will affect your ability to exercise in some way. The extent to which the changes affect you and your baby will:

▸ be different from the extent to which they affect other women and their pregnancies
▸ depend on the type of exercise you are doing
▸ depend on the stage of your pregnancy; for example, early in your pregnancy a high temperature is more threatening to your baby's development than later, whereas backache is usually more of a misery for you late in your pregnancy than early on.

THE HIDDEN CHANGES

The sections that follow are a straightforward account of the physiological changes occurring during pregnancy that will have an impact on your choice of exercise. The account is by no means exhaustive; rather, it is a basic overview written so that you can develop a respect for the limitations pregnancy imposes on exercise and plan your program accordingly. If you want a fuller description of the complex interaction between body systems and exercise and how they affect pregnancy and vice versa, we suggest you consult texts such as *Exercise in Pregnancy* by R. Artall Mittelmark, R. Wiswell and B. Drinkwater.

Cardiac changes

During pregnancy your heart naturally becomes more efficient so that it can meet the increased demand for blood to supply your growing baby as well as you. Your heart pumps faster and your heart rate when you are at rest is higher. The muscle of your heart enlarges so that it can pump more blood with every beat.

IMPLICATIONS FOR EXERCISE

▸ The good news is that you can usually achieve aerobic benefits with a lower increase of heart rate (that is, with less work) than when you were not pregnant. Your heart is already working harder than normal to meet the metabolic demands of your pregnancy, so you are always in a slightly aerobic state during pregnancy.
▸ Your resting heart rate is higher, so your warm-up doesn't need to be as vigorous as before you were pregnant; however, both your warm-up

and your cool-down should be longer and slower than normal.

▶ Because when you are pregnant the range between your resting heart rate and your heart rate during exercise is smaller than when you were not pregnant, you should limit your level of exertion to what you perceive to be 'somewhat to moderately hard'. Because there is no conclusive research currently available about the maximum safe heart rate during pregnancy, it is difficult to give absolute guidelines. It appears best to use an exercising heart-rate range of between 60 and 75 per cent of your maximum heart rate (see Chapter 5 for an explanation of this), coupled with the perceived level of exertion just described.

▶ Reducing the duration and intensity of the exercise is important as pregnancy progresses. Talk to your medical consultant about what is best for you and your baby.

Vascular changes

During pregnancy you have a greater volume of blood circulating in your body. The increase in fluid (plasma) is greater than the increase in red blood cells, so your blood is relatively 'diluted'. This means its ability to carry oxygen around your body is potentially reduced. However, despite this haemodilution, the oxygen supply to your baby is maintained because your heart is pumping more blood each minute (increased cardiac output), and you are breathing more air per minute (increased minute ventilation) than before you were pregnant so that you build up a reserve of oxygen.

A softening of the walls of your veins (see 'Pregnancy Hormone Changes that Affect Exercise' below) also occurs. This potentially allows blood to pool in the veins of your lower legs.

IMPLICATIONS FOR EXERCISE

▶ You need to avoid prolonged standing exercises and keep your legs moving, so blood does not pool in the veins of your legs.

▶ You should change positions slowly so you don't feel dizzy or light-headed.

▶ You need to avoid lying on your back in later pregnancy because the weight of your uterus can press on the large veins returning blood to your heart and may cause dizziness.

▶ You should limit how hard, how long and how often you work out to the levels recommended in the guidelines given in Chapter 3.

▶ You need to LISTEN TO YOUR BODY and work at your own pace.

Respiratory changes

Because each millilitre of your blood cannot carry as much oxygen as before you became pregnant, your respiratory system must work harder to supply oxygen to your organs and to your baby, especially towards the end of your pregnancy. The hormone progesterone causes you to breathe deeper to maintain a sufficient oxygen supply.

In late pregnancy, your uterus presses right up under your diaphragm, so you may find it harder to breathe deeply. You may even feel some rib pain as your ribs flare sideways to accommodate this change.

The normal respiratory system is not heavily taxed by pregnancy, so there's plenty of oxygen in reserve for moderate exercise. However, in late pregnancy, sudden increases in aerobic work to intense levels can leave you feeling breathless.

IMPLICATIONS FOR EXERCISE

▶ To avoid feeling out of breath, you need to limit your work-out to a level of exertion perceived as no greater than 'moderately hard'.
▶ Exercises such as the trunk stretches (Exercise 24), given in the Home Exercise Program for Pregnancy in Part 2, often feel comfortable late in pregnancy because they tend to relieve the rib pressure.

Pregnancy hormonal changes that affect exercise

Hormones (the chemical monitors of your body) cause a wide variety of changes in your body during pregnancy, which are designed to create a suitable environment for the maintenance and development of a healthy baby.

Temperature changes

During pregnancy, your body temperature is reset by the hormone progesterone at 0.5°C higher than normal. Heat is also generated, even while you rest, by the extra work being done by maternal tissues and the metabolic work of growing your baby. If your core temperature remains elevated for extended periods at critical times during the first thirteen weeks of your pregnancy, you may place your baby at risk of developmental defects. Your core temperature should not rise to or remain above 38°C for extended periods. Do not sunbake or use hot baths, saunas or spas because these activities can raise your temperature.

IMPLICATIONS FOR EXERCISE

▶ You need to be careful not to exercise so intensely that your temperature rises above the maximum of 38°C. It is difficult to perceive a changed core temperature until it is already high; however, if you follow the guidelines regarding exercise intensity and duration outlined in this book, your temperature should remain within safe limits.

▶ You should not exercise if you are ill with a fever or exercise in a hot, humid environment because both situations have the potential to raise your core temperature above safe limits.

Simple precautions you can take to limit a rise in body temperature are:

▶ drink water before, during and after exercise (that is, ensure good hydration)
▶ wear loose, light cotton clothing while exercising
▶ exercise in a cool, well-ventilated environment
▶ limit the intensity and duration of your exercise.

Adrenaline response

The normal group of adrenaline hormones released by everyone as they exercise have specific effects during pregnancy:

▶ they can act as a stimulant to your uterus, causing contractions
▶ they normally play a part in directing the blood flow to your working muscles and away from your internal organs during exercise – the uterus is considered one of the organs that may have blood diverted away from it during pregnancy
▶ they help stabilise glucose levels at mild to moderate levels of exercise, but this effect is reduced during strenuous exercise. Your baby may then be at risk of having a low-blood sugar level during your exercise.

IMPLICATIONS FOR EXERCISE

▶ You need to limit your exercise intensity to 'somewhat to moderately hard' and maintain your target heart rate in accordance with the 'Pregnancy Exercise Guidelines' given in Chapter 3.

- You should limit your 'moderately hard' exercise to 15 minutes duration in your work-out (unless you have specific advice from your medical or exercise consultant).

- If you have had a history of miscarriage, you should discuss your intended exercise program with your medical consultant, preferably prior to conception.

Softening of the joints

Pregnancy hormones, including progesterone but particularly relaxin, cause a chemical change to occur in the ligaments of your joints, in your muscle tendons and in other body structures, such as the walls of your veins and intestines. These structures are chemically 'softened'. Relaxin is produced very early in pregnancy and has its peak production at twelve to fourteen weeks. Although it takes some time for relaxin to cause softening of your ligaments and its effects are not usually felt until later in pregnancy, some women complain of discomfort and softening as early as mid-pregnancy.

The pelvis is normally considered a fused bony ring, similar to the skull. However, under the influence of relaxin, a small amount of movement occurs at each of its joints, causing it to become an unstable ring. It is this movement that may cause discomfort at the front or back of your pelvis or pain to radiate into your buttocks as you move. The most obvious signs of pelvic-joint instability are:

- a pregnant waddle
- pain in the hips or buttocks, especially when you have been standing still for a long time; changed positions, such as rolled over or got out of bed; or taken weight on one side of your body when, for example, climbing stairs.

While the prime purpose of relaxin is to soften your pelvic joints so that they are ready for the birth of your baby, its effects may be felt in other joints of your body, especially those that support your body weight. The structures supporting the small joints of your feet, for example, are softened by relaxin. When you add to this the extra weight you are carrying, you can see why your feet may flatten and widen during pregnancy. The result is usually tired, aching feet and difficulty fitting into some of your shoes.

This hormonal softening also affects the walls of your veins and gut. They tend to widen and may contribute to blood pooling in the lower-leg veins when you stand still for long periods of time, and to constipation, heartburn, gastric reflux and indigestion in the gut.

IMPLICATIONS FOR EXERCISE

▶ You need to protect your pelvic joints during every exercise. Their softened state makes them vulnerable to injury. To help protect them during exercise:

- ▶ avoid high-impact exercises or activities
- ▶ limit asymmetrical weight-bearing activities, such as 'step' classes
- ▶ avoid highly choreographed or fast aerobics
- ▶ exercise in shock-absorbing footwear
- ▶ wear low-heeled shoes – preferably ones that are also wide heeled
- ▶ take shorter strides when you walk
- ▶ brace your abdominals and tuck your pelvis under before all movements (as described later in the chapter)
- ▶ strengthen your postural support muscles; that is, your back, hip and abdominal muscles
- ▶ bring your knees together when you change positions.

▶ You should seek advice from your medical or exercise consultant or from a women's health physiotherapist if you have any problems. Most women respond well to individual consultation and so avoid long-term back and pelvic problems.

OTHER ADVICE FOR COMFORT

To avoid blood pooling:

- ▶ limit the time you spend standing still
- ▶ keep your toes and legs moving if you do have to stand for a long period.

To prevent heartburn and indigestion interfering with your exercise:

- ▶ avoid positions where your shoulders are lower than your hips
- ▶ take frequent small sips of water during exercise.

To help relieve constipation:

▶ eat a well-balanced diet rich in fibre and drink plenty of water
▶ practise pelvic rocking – some women find it helps relieve bowel discomfort.

To protect your feet:

▶ as mentioned above, wear supportive low, wide-heeled shoes as much as possible and exercise in shock-absorbing footwear
▶ avoid constant walking on concrete when walking for exercise
▶ consider being fitted with orthotics by a podiatrist.

'Packaging problems'

All pregnant women experience some discomfort from the compression and stretching associated with the growing uterus. Before you were pregnant, your uterus was much smaller than the size of your fist. By the end of your pregnancy it will be about the size of a punching bag – and that's if you're having only one baby! The packaging of the structures within your abdomen will obviously need to be rearranged to accommodate this growth.

Effects on the rib cage

Towards the end of pregnancy, your uterus will press up under your diaphragm. The work of breathing will become harder, especially during moderate to high-intensity exercise. You will feel short of breath more easily. To compensate for the limitations of your diaphragm, your ribs will flare out to the side as you breathe, which may cause a sharp pain under your shoulder blades that radiates to your chest.

IMPLICATIONS FOR EXERCISE

▶ You will need to avoid moderate to high-intensity exercise during the last trimester of pregnancy.
▶ You should avoid sudden changes of aerobic intensity in your exercise program – sustained, light to moderate aerobic work is preferable.
▶ You should add upper-back flexibility exercises to reduce the risk of rib pain.

• You should seek physiotherapy treatment if rib pain is a persistent problem.

Pelvic-floor pressure

The pelvic floor is the group of muscles that attach in a hammock-like fashion to the base of your pelvis. An important function of these muscles is to support the abdominal and pelvic contents above them, including your bladder and uterus.

The design of the pelvic floor is considered inherently poor because, firstly, the group of muscles that form the pelvic floor have only a small amount of muscle fibre, but a large amount of fibrous tissue and, secondly, they are interrupted by the urethra, vagina and anus. Maybe the pelvic floor wasn't designed to take all the weight from above at all? Perhaps we were designed to walk around on all fours as the theory of evolution suggests!

During pregnancy, there is an increased risk of incontinence (involuntary loss of urine). The three major contributing factors are:

1 the increased pressure on your bladder and pelvic floor as your uterus expands
2 the increasing amount of space your uterus occupies within the pelvis as your pregnancy progresses, which makes it impossible for your bladder to hold as much urine as before
3 the hormone relaxin, which softens the structures of the pelvic floor so that they become less efficient in holding up your pelvic organs. This can also add to the discomfort of vulval varicose veins and haemorrhoids.

When you pull, push, lift or carry loads, cough, sneeze, vomit, run, jump or laugh heartily you increase the pressure within your abdomen, which will jeopardise an already 'at risk' situation even further. The pelvic-floor muscles may not be able to hold against this extra pressure and stress incontinence may be the consequence. (Stress incontinence is the involuntary leakage of urine caused by an increase in impact or stress pressure within the abdomen.) The best defence you have is to avoid situations that place added strain on your body and to improve the strength of your pelvic-floor muscles.

If you find that you have some degree of incontinence when you cough, sneeze, laugh, lift, push, pull, run, jump, walk fast or, in fact, do any other activity, you should:

▶ strictly practise and increase your repetitions of the exercises given in 'Pelvic-floor Bracing' below
▶ seek professional treatment.

PELVIC-FLOOR BRACING

For everyday protection against the effects of gravity and the increasing weight of your uterus during pregnancy, you need to improve the holding (isometric) tone of your pelvic-floor muscles. To fully strengthen your pelvic floor you should do the following exercises often throughout the day.

Bracing

Imagine yourself tightening around your urethra, vagina and anus, then lift up internally, hold the position for a few seconds (without holding your breath) and then release it slowly. Repeat the exercise several times. To improve the strength of your pelvic-floor muscles, aim gradually to increase the length of your hold and the number of repetitions that you do. Hold this brace and lift in all your upright postures and especially when there is increasing pressure on the muscles from above as, for example, when you lift, cough or sneeze. During most of the exercises given in Parts 2 and 3, hold your pelvic-floor muscles gently braced by tightening around your urethra, vagina and anus.

Lift, Release, Lift, Release

This is a short hold, followed by a rest of the same length, done repetitively to help strengthen the pelvic-floor muscles required when you cough or sneeze suddenly.

IMPLICATIONS FOR EXERCISE

▶ You need to develop a pelvic-floor strengthening regime that becomes a part of your daily life. This is the best way to minimise the impact of pregnancy on your pelvic floor. Even if you were already practising pelvic-floor exercises daily before you became pregnant, you will need to work at them harder during pregnancy.

▶ You can reduce the risk of stress incontinence when you exercise by:

   ▶ avoiding high-impact activities, such as running, jumping and bouncing

   ▶ bracing your pelvic-floor muscles before you do any sit-up style of exercise or any lifting or resistance work with weights because of the increased intra-abdominal pressure during these exercises

   ▶ being aware of tightening, or bracing, your pelvic-floor muscles during all upright exercises.

TIP FOR BIRTH READINESS

During birth your pelvic-floor muscles will act as a guide for your baby's passage through the birth canal, so in addition to strengthening your pelvic-floor muscles also spend some time releasing the muscles fully. In late pregnancy when you are relaxing each day, imagine letting go of all pelvic-floor muscle tension and making a passage for your baby through your pelvic outlet. This exercise can also be done in practice birth positions, such as hands and knees, side-lying and standing supported squats. Make sure you tighten your pelvic-floor muscles again afterwards.

THE OBVIOUS CHANGES

The more obvious changes of pregnancy are those that relate to the external changes in the shape of a woman's body. By the twelfth week of pregnancy your baby (foetus) should have developed all its major organs. From then until birth it should continue to grow and mature within your uterus.

As your baby grows during pregnancy, your uterus will outgrow the space it normally occupies within your pelvis and move up into your abdomen, pressing on other structures as it does so. The top (fundus) of your uterus is usually just above your pubic bone by about twelve weeks, and level with your bellybutton by twenty weeks. While each pregnancy is different, you will usually begin to 'show' during this time and may start to feel your baby move. Once the uterus is 'showing' there may be a greater risk of falling and trauma during some exercise.

Most women experience breast changes from early pregnancy. The breasts usually become larger and feel fuller as pregnancy progresses, which may make some forms of exercise uncomfortable.

The pattern and timing of weight gained in pregnancy varies. In addition to the changes in your breasts and abdomen, you will probably notice changes around your buttocks and thighs, and even your face. If you are eating a well-balanced diet of adequate amount and exercising regularly you will need to accept your changing shape as a natural expression of your pregnancy.

Postural adjustments

Your change in posture will become obvious to all. As the size of your baby increases, your centre of gravity will move forward to in front of your hips, causing your pelvis to tip forward. The curve of your spine will increase (your lower back will become more swayed and your shoulders rounded) to compensate for this and to maintain your balance. If you remember the line

Maintaining a balanced posture during exercise will help reduce the risk of back and pelvic discomfort.

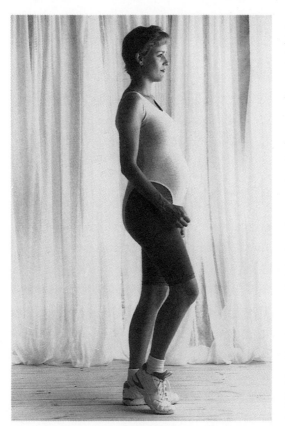

from the old song, 'Your knee bone's connected to your thigh bone . . .', you will understand that when there is a change in one part of your posture, there are compensatory adjustments throughout your body, particularly in your spine.

During pregnancy your posture will be constantly adjusting to accommodate your baby's growth, so you will need to be vigilant about finding your best balanced posture. As you move from one position to another (for example, when you get out of bed) consider how you hold your pelvis and remember to brace your abdominal muscles to balance your spinal posture.

Achieving balanced posture

- ▶ Extend your neck and spine as if you were balancing a book on your head.
- ▶ When standing, have your knees 'soft' rather than locked. This will allow you to hold your pelvis tilted to a comfortably 'flat-backed' position rather than the sway-backed position common in pregnancy.
- ▶ Feel 'open' across your chest: bring your shoulder blades together by gently bracing the muscles between them, but keep your shoulders relaxed.
- ▶ Hold your abdominal and pelvic-floor muscles gently braced, as described in this chapter.

If you leave your posture unchecked in pregnancy, the forward drag on your spinal and pelvic joints due to your increased weight and altered centre of gravity may lead to lower-back and pelvic pain developing. The abdominal strengthening and pelvic-mobility exercises described in this book have been specially chosen to help you maintain a balanced posture in all positions and so help prevent back discomfort and pelvic-joint strain.

IMPLICATIONS FOR EXERCISE

- ▶ You need to be diligent in maintaining your balanced posture in all positions and exercises.
- ▶ You should make sure you strengthen your abdominal and buttock muscles so that you can control your pelvic tilt as your pregnancy progresses.
- ▶ You need to support and protect your pelvic and spinal joints by using pelvic-floor and abdominal-bracing techniques throughout all exercises.
- ▶ You should 'think tall' at all times.

Stretched abdominal muscles

The abdominal muscles act as a natural 'corset' to support your abdominal organs and to produce the movement of your spine and pelvis. This

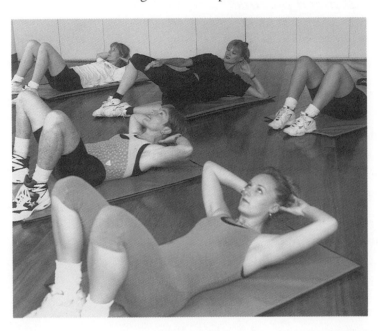

corset is elastic and made up of different layers of muscles (rectus, oblique and transverse fibres) crossing each other to increase the strength of the corset as well as to produce the movements of your trunk. The right and left abdominal-muscle groups are joined at the front with a central fibrous structure known as the linea alba. This is the corset's point of weakness.

As your baby grows within your uterus, your abdominal muscles will have to stretch to accommodate this growth. The linea alba may naturally give way if it is under too much pressure, rather than allow the abdominal-muscle fibres to overstretch or tear. Known as diastasis (diastasis recti abdominis), this separation should be considered a safety feature rather than a dramatic injury. If you look after your abdominals during pregnancy and the early days after childbirth, this separation should naturally resolve itself within six to eight weeks after the birth.

As your pregnancy progresses, you will need to change from abdominal curl-ups on your back to an alternative position.

Whenever you pull, push or lift or sit up from a lying position, the pressure within your abdomen increases. The thinned or separated fibrous tissue of the linea alba may not be able to withstand this build-up of abdominal pressure. Bulging, or herniation, may occur along the central line of your abdomen. This is an indication that the weight or resistance is too heavy for you, so:

▶ take care with your abdominal exercises, with transferring from one position to another, such as moving from a lying position to the upright position, and when you are lifting, pushing or carrying things
▶ remember that heavy lifting during pregnancy is not recommended.

The abdominal sit-ups, or 'crunches', that you may have done prior to pregnancy become ineffective and inappropriate during pregnancy — ineffective because of the stretch on your abdominal muscles (the muscles cannot work the way they did before you were pregnant); and inappropriate because lying on your back as your pregnancy progresses means the weight of the growing uterus will rest on the major blood vessels in front of your spine, which may decrease the return of blood to your heart (supine hypotension).

As your pregnancy progresses and your centre of gravity shifts forward, your abdominal muscles must carry an ever-increasing load. Their ability to support this load is dependent on their tone or strength. If your abdominals are weak, they will not be able to support your spine adequately. The result will be increasing back and pelvic discomfort or pain. So *work your front (abdominals) to protect your back!* Backache and pelvic-joint discomfort can also be relieved by lowering your centre of gravity and widening your base of support. Being on their hands and knees is a very comfortable resting position for many women in late pregnancy.

IMPLICATIONS FOR EXERCISE

▶ To protect your abdominals, you should replace traditional curl-ups done in the supine position (lying on your back) with the postural techniques given in 'Abdominal Bracing: "Press-studs", Waistline Gathering and Pelvic Tucks' below. Also use the alternative strengthening exercises, and the techniques for transferring from one position to the next, given in the Home Exercise Program for Pregnancy in Part 2 (see Exercises 14, and 18 to 20). This may reduce the potential for diastasis during pregnancy and help it to settle naturally within six to eight weeks after childbirth.

▶ It is important that you continue to breathe comfortably throughout your exercises so that you do not increase the pressure within your abdomen unnecessarily. Increased intra-abdominal pressure puts more strain on the abdominal fibrous junction.

▶ Use any of the postural abdominal exercises that follow when doing the exercises described in the Home Exercise Program for Pregnancy. This way you will maximise the tone and strength developed in your abdominals and protect yourself from injury because you are supporting your spine while you do other movements.

ABDOMINAL BRACING: 'PRESS-STUDS', WAISTLINE GATHERING AND PELVIC TUCKS

Postural abdominal exercises, also known as bracing, are sometimes more difficult than they seem. Take your time and practise them often until they become automatic. Eventually you should be able to hold your abdominal muscles braced and your pelvis tucked in throughout the day, while breathing comfortably.

'Press-studs'

Imagine pressing your bellybutton internally through to your spine as if you were doing up a press-stud or Velcro fastening, then hold this position.

Waistline gathering

Imagine you want to wear your belt on the next smallest hole. Pull your waist in all the way round and hold this position comfortably, remembering to breathe easily; or imagine you are able to give your baby a hug within your pelvis – feel yourself wrapping your 'arms' (your abdominal muscles) all the way round the baby.

Pelvic tucks

Imagine that your pelvis is a bassinette, and lift your baby up and in towards your spine, placing him or her back securely into the carriage of your pelvis; or imagine you have a searchlight attached to your bellybutton, and make the light search a long way ahead rather than at your feet. You should feel tight around your tummy as you hold this pelvic tuck; however, be reassured that you cannot squash your baby by doing these exercises.

The advantages of these exercises in pregnancy are that they:

▶ can be done throughout the day
▶ can be done throughout your pregnancy
▶ will help prevent or relieve back and pelvic pain.

ADVICE ON ABDOMINAL SEPARATION

To help prevent the bulging of abdominal separation:

▶ do pelvic tucks before any exercise that builds up intra-abdominal pressure (for example, any resistance work)
▶ brace your abdominal muscles, using the techniques described opposite, before changing positions during exercise – and at any time
▶ use the postural exercises given above and the pelvic-rocking exercises (Exercises 3, 14 and 18) given in the Home Exercise Program for Pregnancy in Part 2, rather than traditional curl-up exercises, for your abdominal-strengthening exercises.

TIP

The best position for strengthening your abdominal muscles during late pregnancy is on your hands and knees, and the best exercise in this position is pelvic rocking (see Exercise 14 given in the Home Exercise Program for Pregnancy in Part 2).

guidelines for minimising risks

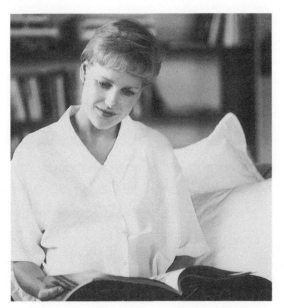

Exercising in pregnancy means making choices for two people: you and your baby. Your exercise should be different during pregnancy from other times in your life, and needs to balance your personal goals with the needs of your developing baby.

While your level of exercise during pregnancy generally reflects your previous exercise experience, the health of your pregnancy and your comfort may override this. You may be someone who exercised regularly before pregnancy, but your medical consultant has advised you to rest for the early part of your pregnancy because of your history of several miscarriages; or you may be an athlete who has no problems with the health of the pregnancy, and so find you are able, by modifying your program, to continue your training through most of your pregnancy until the size or weight of your baby forces you to stop; or you may be a sportswoman who is not having any problems with the health of the pregnancy, but you are just finding the nausea and fatigue of early pregnancy difficult and you are not enjoying your previous exercise choices any more!

Irrespective of previous exercise experience, one of the most common questions asked is 'Is exercise safe during pregnancy?'. In general, provided you are healthy, you can assume that exercise is safe if:

▶ your pregnancy progresses normally
▶ you seek regular advice from your medical consultant
▶ you are prepared to change your exercise as your pregnancy progresses.

Even if you have exercised regularly for years, you need to learn to listen to your body and your baby, and give yourself permission to slow down during pregnancy as required. And if you haven't done any exercise for ages, now may be a good time to think about starting a special program!

SEEKING ADVICE

It is important that you seek advice about what exercise to do during pregnancy. Discuss your exercise needs with your medical or exercise consultant, who can help design an exercise program suitable for you and your baby. The factors you and your consultant need to consider when choosing include your health and your baby's, and your previous experience of exercise, as discussed in the following sections. And, as a pregnant woman who wants to exercise, you will need to be aware of, and seek advice about, the risks involved in your choice of exercise and the symptoms that may signal a need to stop or change your exercise, which are outlined later in the chapter.

YOUR AND YOUR BABY'S HEALTH

When considering your health and your baby's, take note that there are some medical conditions that will preclude you from exercising. These are listed in 'Medical Conditions and Exercise' below. Your medical consultant will screen you for these conditions at your prenatal visits. As well, there are some conditions (also listed) that may preclude you from certain types of exercise, depending on:

- ▶ the frequency, intensity, duration and type of exercise you wish to undertake
- ▶ the environment in which you exercise
- ▶ your experience of that exercise.

There are very few women who need to stop exercising completely during pregnancy. With the right advice and support, you may still be able to do something. It is important that you tell your medical consultant if you change your exercise program so you can be advised accordingly. It is also important to keep your exercise consultant, if you have one, up to date with the developments in your pregnancy.

YOUR PREVIOUS EXPERIENCE OF EXERCISE

Being careful with the way you move during your exercise session will help prevent unnecessary strain.

The type and amount of exercise you participated in before pregnancy will generally influence the type and amount of exercise that is safe for your developing baby and for your own body. When you exercise regularly, your body adapts well to the physiological changes of exercise. Your heart can

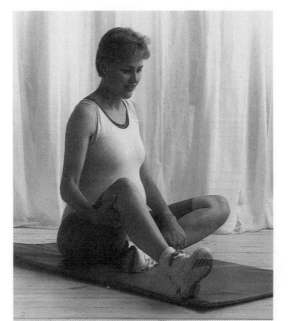

pump more efficiently, your body's control of temperature changes is better, and so on. Because of these adaptations some women who are experienced exercisers appear to be able to exercise more vigorously during pregnancy than women just starting out. However, take care, as this is not always the case.

If you haven't exercised regularly for a while, pregnancy can be a good time to start a specially designed exercise program, after seeking advice. Exercise can make you feel more comfortable during your pregnancy and better prepared for the extra physical effort associated with having and caring for a new baby.

Medical conditions and exercise

The two lists that follow include the medical conditions that the American College of Obstetricians and Gynecologists considers preclude or may preclude your exercising during pregnancy.

Medical conditions that preclude exercise

These medical conditions *will generally* preclude your exercising during pregnancy:

- heart disease
- thrombophlebitis
- recent pulmonary embolism
- acute infectious disease
- uterine bleeding or ruptured membranes
- risk of premature labour
- incompetent cervix
- intra-uterine growth retardation
- severe iso-immunisation
- severe high blood pressure
- multiple pregnancy (triplets or more)
- suspected foetal distress
- placenta praevia
- no prenatal care.

Medical conditions that may preclude exercise

These medical conditions *may* preclude your exercising or require you to change your choice of exercise:

- anaemia or other blood disorders
- high blood pressure
- thyroid disease
- diabetes mellitus
- multiple pregnancy (twins)
- breech presentation in the last trimester
- excessively over or under weight
- history of sedentary lifestyle.

Remember

- Your health, and your baby's, will continue to influence what exercise is right, throughout your pregnancy.
- Your exercise should reflect your experience.
- Your exercise may need to change as your pregnancy progresses.
- You should not compare yourself directly with other women, or this pregnancy with other pregnancies you have had.
- If you have been involved in competitive sport, you may need to reduce your training, and it is generally recommended that you reduce your level of competition.

RISKY EXERCISE CHOICES

There are some forms of exercise that just aren't worth the risk when you are pregnant. These include:

- activities and sports where there is a risk of collision, tripping or falling or heavy body contact
- team competition where you have to reach, stretch or leap beyond the safe limits for your joints and your baby
- activities that take place in an unsafe environment, such as air or water at high temperatures, or those that use heavy equipment or equipment likely to cause heavy contact
- exercises or sports where the 'adrenaline rush' you get from the competitiveness or the nature of the exercise or sport overrides your common sense — even sports that are theoretically suitable during pregnancy may become unsuitable due to your personal competitiveness
- activities involving repetitive high impact, lots of twists and turns, high stepping or sudden stops, which may cause joint discomfort.

It is therefore not recommended that you:

- parachute
- bungee jump
- water ski or snow ski
- scuba dive or board dive

- be involved in dance or choreography where performance or group movement carries you past the point of safety
- ride horses or do any activity where there is a risk of falling
- play any team game or be involved in competition activities where winning is of major importance. When considering competition, ask your sports association and your coach about the local regulations governing pregnant women competing in that sport.

While activities such as running, netball, aerobics and squash are not banned in pregnancy, you should critically assess their suitability for you. It may be better as your pregnancy progresses to consider alternatives that will still allow you to maintain your fitness.

Remember   If in doubt, ASK!

WARNING SIGNS

Listed below are the signals that will tell you if your body is not coping with the level of exercise you have chosen. Stop exercising and seek advice from your medical or exercise consultant if any of the following occur:

- pain of any kind (the most likely musculo-skeletal pains are in the back, pelvis or hip) – do *not* push through this pain
- discomfort after your exercise session
- difficulty in walking or moving during or after the exercise session
- contractions of your uterus at 15-minute intervals or less – these may be experienced as abdominal cramps or back pain
- vaginal bleeding or leaking of amniotic fluid
- dizziness or faintness
- headaches or visual disturbances
- generalised swelling
- numbness in any part of the body
- persistent fatigue
- nausea or vomiting
- slow or reducing weight gain
- decreased movements of your baby.

Be alert for these signs at any stage of your pregnancy. Remember to regularly consult your medical consultant about the continued suitability of exercise as your pregnancy progresses. Always be prepared to change your exercise program as required.

As you exercise, you may experience some signals that indicate you need to change your exercise program. The following are examples of relatively common problems that can be managed either by you or with help.

Supine and postural hypotension

When you lie on your back, stand still for too long or change positions too quickly, you may feel dizzy, light-headed or even faint. This is due to a decrease in the blood being returned to your heart and brain.

ADVICE

▸ Change positions more slowly.
▸ Use central or stabilising postures during position changes.
▸ Avoid lying on your back from about the sixteenth week of pregnancy.
▸ Avoid prolonged standing without movement.
▸ Roll onto your side to restore the blood flow.

Overheating

Overheating of your body may change the environment within your uterus, causing heat stress for your baby as well as distress for you. Early symptoms of overheating are headache, light-headedness and nausea. The more advanced signs are chills, unsteadiness and clammy skin, and medical attention may be required.

ADVICE

▸ Limit the duration and intensity of your exercise.
▸ Keep well hydrated by drinking water during your exercise.
▸ Exercise in a cool and well-ventilated environment.
▸ Don't exercise in high humidity.
▸ Don't exercise if you have a high temperature.
▸ Wear loose, light clothing made of natural fibre.

FIRST AID FOR OVERHEATING

Cool your body by:

▸ stopping your exercise and resting in a cool place
▸ exposing your skin to the air by taking off some clothes

- drinking some cool or cold water
- keeping air moving over your skin, using a fan.

Low blood sugar

As your pregnancy progresses, your energy (glucose) needs increase. Your body needs more fuel just for growing your baby. Exercise uses glucose for muscle fuel, and this can further reduce your body's glucose stores, so you may need to eat more to increase your energy. In late pregnancy, you may feel hungry all the time. LISTEN TO YOUR BODY and eat enough (healthy choices, of course) to provide fuel for your baby's growth and for your exercise. Symptoms of low blood sugar (hypoglycaemia) include drowsiness, apathy, irritability, hand tremors, poor co-ordination, visual disturbances, dizziness and headaches.

ADVICE

- Eat a complex-carbohydrate snack one to two hours before exercising (for example, a piece of fruit or a bread product).
- If you are experiencing the symptoms of hypoglycaemia regularly, have a sugar snack on hand when you exercise (for example, orange juice or jelly beans).
- It's wise to have your next snack or meal within an hour of exercise to replenish your fuel losses.
- Stop exercising and rest.
- Review your exercise program. You may need to reduce your exercise intensity or duration.
- Seek advice from your medical consultant if these solutions do not reduce the symptoms or they happen regularly. You may also need to consult a dietician.

Note If your hypoglycaemia is associated with either gestational diabetes or diabetes mellitus, regular exercise under supervision can help regulate your blood-glucose levels.

Pelvic-joint pain

The normally immovable pelvic joints are softened by the pregnancy hormones and there is potential for movement at these joints. Movement may occur at the front of your pelvis at the pubic joint, or at the back of your pelvis at the sacro-iliac joints. Pain around these joints or radiating into your hips, groin or buttocks is an indication that the pelvic ring is becoming unstable. Pelvic-joint pain is most often felt when you:

- start to move; that is, as you lift your leg
- change positions; for example, when you roll over in bed
- stand or walk for long periods, especially on concrete; for example, when you are out shopping
- use repetitive asymmetrical or unilateral movements in activities such as climbing stairs, vacuuming or doing step classes.

Remember   Pelvic-joint pain is often felt after you finish your activity or exercise rather than during it.

ADVICE

- The simplest, age-old remedy is gentle pelvic rocking within the limits of your pain. This is best done leaning forward to take the weight off your pelvic joints (see Exercise 14 given in the Home Exercise Program for Pregnancy in Part 2).
- From the hands and knees position, sit back on your heels and lean forward to stretch the region and hence relieve pain (see Exercise 17 in Part 2).
- Walk more slowly and shorten your stride.
- Strengthen your abdominal and pelvic-floor muscles to help support the weight of your baby, so there is less drag on your pelvic joints.
- Lie on your side with your knees bent up and resting on top of each other. This is also a good sleeping position, with or without a pillow between your knees.

Threat of premature labour

Signals of premature labour include:

- regular lower-back pains or menstrual-like cramps that are getting stronger and closer together
- bowel cramps, with or without diarrhoea
- pressure in the lower abdomen, back or thighs
- vaginal discharge of either blood or fluid.

ADVICE

▸ Stop exercising immediately.
▸ Make the necessary phone calls to your medical consultant and hospital.
▸ Rest while assistance arrives.

Pre-eclampsia

Pre-eclampsia, or toxaemia of pregnancy, is a condition that can develop from mid-pregnancy onwards and may develop gradually or suddenly. If it goes untreated, it can be life-threatening and may require the immediate delivery of your baby. Signs of pre-eclampsia include:

▸ high blood pressure
▸ swelling of your hands, feet, neck and face that does not go away
▸ headaches and visual disturbances
▸ protein in your urine (tested at your antenatal visits).

ADVICE

If you notice any combination of the signs above, seek your medical consultant's advice before contemplating any activity, including walking the dog or going shopping.

Remember For your own and your baby's safety, before participating in exercise during pregnancy you should consult your medical consultant. Seeking advice from an exercise consultant will help you design a tailor-made program. The information in this book is of a general nature and does not replace the need for individual advice.

PREGNANCY EXERCISE GUIDELINES

On the basis of the information currently available, we suggest you observe the following guidelines for exercise during pregnancy.

1   Your core temperature should not rise above 38°C. To keep within a safe temperature range, reduce your exercise intensity and keep well hydrated by drinking water during your exercise. Do not exercise if you are already ill with a high temperature or if the weather is hot and humid, and do not sunbake or have hot saunas, baths or spas.

2   The vigorous component of your exercise program should not exceed 15 minutes, unless you are an experienced exerciser and you are advised otherwise by your medical or exercise consultant.

3   Your perceived level of exertion should be limited to a level you would describe as 'somewhat to moderately hard'. If you are used to calculating your heart rate to determine the intensity of your work-out (see Chapter 5), a target exercise heart-rate range of between 60 and 75 per cent of your maximum heart rate is adequate. Your heart rate should not exceed 140 beats per minute unless you seek advice from your medical or exercise consultant. (Obviously you do not have to reach these upper limits if you already feel you are exercising within your comfortable range.)

4   If you have not done much regular physical activity prior to your pregnancy, you should begin with activities of low intensity and gradually advance. You should aim to be active three or four times a week. Your exercise should feel comfortable.

5   Choose a variety of aerobic activities (see Chapter 5) to alter the stresses on your body.

6   Have a longer time for warm-up and cool-down to allow for the cardiovascular changes associated with pregnancy. It is also important not to stop your exercise suddenly as this can cause blood pooling in the legs, low blood pressure and possible fainting.

7   It is safer not to lie on your back for long once the bulk of your uterus is within your abdomen as the size and weight of your uterus and baby can partially occlude blood flow returning to the heart. Your abdominal muscles can be strengthened effectively in many other positions.

8   Participate in low-impact exercise to limit the potential of injury to the ligaments and muscles affected by the hormonal changes of pregnancy. Asymmetrical or unilateral activities, such as step classes and rapidly changing choreography, may also stress pelvic joints. Pelvic-joint instability may not always be noticed as pain during the activity, but as a seemingly unrelated pain hours later.

9   To provide adequate energy for your pregnancy and your exercise, adjust your intake of kilojoules by increasing your intake of foods rich in complex carbohydrates, such as breads, cereals, fruit and vegetables.

10   Eat a complex-carbohydrate snack, such as a piece of fruit or a bread product, one to two hours before exercising. To replenish your fuel and to avoid fatigue, it's wise to have your next snack or meal within an hour of exercising.

11   Drink plenty of fluid before, during and after exercise to maintain your hydration.

12   In the gym, reduce weights by approximately 20 to 25 per cent to allow for the load of pregnancy. You should be able to comfortably lift ten to fifteen repetitions of your chosen load. In other words, concentrate on endurance rather than strength gains during pregnancy.

13   Exercise should be modified to suit your pregnancy, and it should take into account the continual changes of posture in pregnancy that affect a pregnant woman's ability to perform some exercises.

14   Stop exercising and seek appropriate advice if any pain or unusual symptoms occur during or after exercise.

designing a safe exercise program

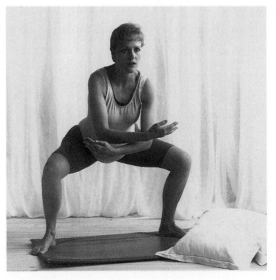

Now that you've sought advice and found that there is no medical reason for you not to exercise, you will need ask yourself, 'What do I want to achieve from my exercise?'. The reasons why women want to exercise vary, depending on their previous experience and enjoyment of exercise. Some of the most common reasons given for exercising in pregnancy are to control weight gain, to prepare for childbirth and to maintain fitness.

CONTROLLING WEIGHT GAIN

Most medical consultants recommend a weight gain of 10 to 12 kilograms in pregnancy. Some women will put on more, others less, and still have a healthy-sized baby and not have gained excessive weight themselves. We are all different. The key is a balance between your energy needs, your baby's and the amount of kilojoules you consume.

The weight you gain during pregnancy will be made up of extra circulating blood, larger breasts, extra muscle and fat and, of course, your baby, uterus, placenta and amniotic fluid. It is the distribution of the extra fat on hips and thighs that causes some women to be very concerned about their weight gain, particularly if they do not understand that this weight distribution is normal and is caused by the hormones of pregnancy.

Excessive weight gain in pregnancy is not recommended because this puts extra strain on your body and can lead to physical discomfort for you and a less than optimal environment for your baby. Controlling excessive weight gain by diet and exercise is therefore a healthy alternative. Research has shown that the best exercise for anyone, pregnant or not, wishing to control their weight is mild to moderate aerobic exercise, maintained over an extended time. This is also an ideal type of exercise during pregnancy as it complies with the guidelines given in Chapter 3. Walking and swimming are probably the most common forms of aerobic exercise used by pregnant women; the other types of aerobic activities available are discussed in Chapter 5.

Make sure controlling excessive weight gain remains your aim with your program and don't become obsessive. Exercising in order not to gain weight at all tips the balance to unhealthy exercise. If you are concerned about your weight gain during pregnancy or whether your diet is adequate nutritionally for the demands of both pregnancy and exercise, you may wish to consult a dietician.

PREPARING FOR CHILDBIRTH

Labour is a very physical event, an event that requires you to have both endurance and strength. If you enter this event physically prepared, your ability to handle it will be enhanced. Just as no sensible athlete would ever consider entering an endurance event without suitable training, adequate rest and appropriate diet, neither should you. Suitable training for childbirth aims to make you strong and flexible, both in body and mind, and to give you specific skills and movements such as pelvic rocking for use during labour.

The Home Exercise Program for Pregnancy in Part 2 is ideal as a preparation for childbirth. Physical strength and flexibility can be gained from the exercises, and mental preparation from the relaxation time you spend at the end of each session as you become in tune with your body and your baby. It can be used on its own or as a complement to other general fitness activities.

MAINTAINING FITNESS

General fitness is most often defined in terms of an improvement in stamina, strength and flexibility. While this definition is still relevant for pregnancy and for new mothers, we at Changing Shape believe a better working definition of fitness is: '*You have enough energy to do your normal daily tasks and have enough left over for the "extras" of life, whether they be social activities, emergency demands or the birth of your baby*'.

Having more energy than you need for the basic tasks of life means that you are not always feeling stretched just to complete these tasks, and that your body is functioning without undue stress being placed on your muscles, joints and body organs.

Fitness levels are specific to each individual so, rather than comparing yourself with other women, you need to be in tune with your own body and aware of your special needs. It is important to recognise the signs your body gives you about its level of fitness and its coping ability, namely:

▶ PAIN – a signal to stop or slow down
▶ BREATHLESSNESS – a signal to slow down and listen for other signs.

COMPONENTS OF A FITNESS PLAN

A working definition of fitness gives you an overall picture, but it's also important to consider the specific components of fitness so you can create a fitness plan to suit your needs. An exercise program that balances aerobic fitness (stamina), strength and flexibility with specific pregnancy skills is ideal for pregnancy.

Aerobic fitness

When you are aerobically fit, you can achieve more with less fatigue; that is, you have that 'extra energy in my day' feeling – that sense of more energy in reserve, more endurance. To develop aerobic fitness, whole body movements are used to increase your heart rate to a prescribed level (your target heart rate, which measures the *intensity* of your exercise, as discussed further in Chapter 5) and to maintain this for a set length of time (the *duration* of your exercise) to improve your heart and lung efficiency.

During pregnancy, your vigorous aerobic work-out will need to last approximately 15 minutes exercising at a moderate intensity to gain aerobic benefits without risk to your baby. Remember to balance the two factors of exercise intensity and duration. If you work out at a higher intensity, you may need to

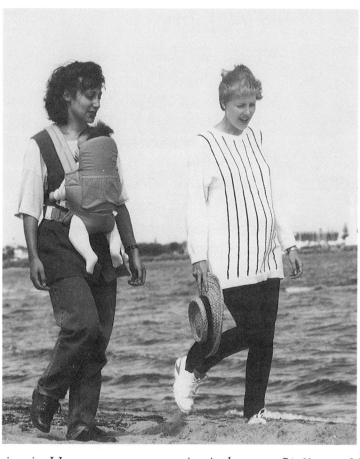

Walking with friends is a great way to enjoy aerobic fitness.

reduce the time you spend doing it. However, you can maintain lower-intensity aerobic exercise, such as walking, for a longer time.

Strength

To develop strength and an ability to lift, carry, push and pull, muscles need to work against a resistance, such as gravity, water or weights. When your muscles are strong, you are more able to resist forces that might otherwise cause injury. You will have better muscle tone and posture and you can carry heavier loads, such as the load of pregnancy or a new baby, more comfortably.

To strengthen your muscles efficiently when you exercise:

▶ tighten, or set, your muscles before you use them in an exercise
▶ move smoothly and at a steady pace through the movement
▶ go right to the end of your range of movement for each exercise
▶ at the end of each exercise hold the position for a moment before returning to your starting position.

Flexibility

To increase your suppleness and flexibility, joints should be worked through their full range of movement and muscles need to be stretched. When you are flexible, you move with ease and are more comfortable in new positions, such as squatting. You will move more gracefully and have better posture and muscle balance, and you will be at less risk of joint or muscle injury.

Flexibility is best achieved by stretches after your body has been thoroughly warmed. Move your limb into the stretch slowly and easily and, when the end of the range is reached, hold this position for 6 to 20 seconds, depending on the aim of the stretch.

Endurance

Having good endurance means that your muscles can work for a longer period of time without becoming fatigued. Aerobic endurance and muscular endurance are both necessary for complete fitness. The advantage of having a good level of endurance is you have the ability to complete a task; to hold or carry a load for longer; and to manage better the physical demands of labour and mothering.

Postural awareness

Postural awareness involves more than just having the strength and flexibility to hold yourself erect. It includes a sense of your position and balance, of knowing where your body is in space. Postural awareness also involves economy of movement, breathing awareness and good alignment during all your movements. The changes in your posture caused by your weight being carried more to the front each month make postural awareness especially hard to maintain as pregnancy progresses. You need to develop strength in your abdominal and back muscles and consciously train yourself to find your best balanced posture (see Chapter 2).

Rest and recovery

Rest is needed for your body to physiologically replenish itself and for recovery from exercise. Recent research indicates that the recovery time between exercise sessions is an important factor in the healthy development of your baby. You need to be aware that the metabolic demands on your body in growing a baby do increase as the nine months of pregnancy progress, so rest and recovery become even more important in the later stages of pregnancy. Rest and recovery take time. If you listen to your body and allow time for rest, you will be rewarded with extra vitality, a feeling of wellbeing, and a lessened risk of injury.

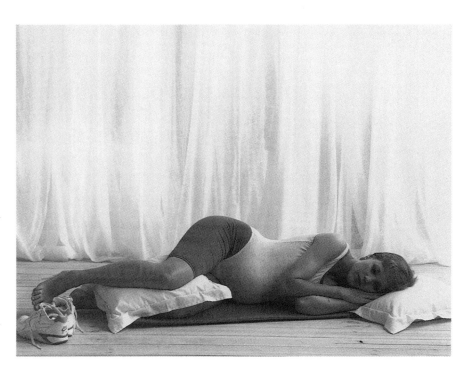

Note   For your and your baby's health, three or four aerobic exercise sessions per week on alternate days are considered ideal during pregnancy.

Allowing time for rest during pregnancy is important for your baby's health and your wellbeing.

Specific pregnancy exercise

Childbirth is a physical event, and exercise is essential to prepare for labour and for recovery afterwards. Compared with those of women in previous generations, our bodies are generally not work-hardened. We don't have to scrub floors on our hands and knees or walk long distances carrying our shopping. Therefore today we need to develop the endurance to cope physically with labour through regular exercise.

If you are hoping to be upright and active during your labour, you will need to develop specific fitness skills to help you do so. In addition to being generally fit you will need to learn skills such as:

▶ improving the flexibility of your lower back and your hips so that you can change positions easily

▶ strengthening your hip and buttock muscles so you can achieve the wide open pelvic positions, such as deep squatting, which are often comfortable in labour

▶ tightening and relaxing your pelvic floor so that you can be aware of your baby passing through your birth canal during labour

- pelvic rocking in different positions for pain relief during contractions
- breathing control during all your exercises to focus and conserve energy.

WHAT TYPE OF EXERCISE IS BEST?

The importance of each of the above components of fitness for you will depend on:

- your previous experience of exercise
- your own aims in exercising
- which fitness components you feel need most practice.

Use the following scenarios to help you decide what weight you might give to the components of fitness during your pregnancy.

I work out at the gym three times per week and swim weekly . . .
Congratulations! You have already established the good habit of regular exercise.

What should you focus on?
- Understand your body changes and how they will affect your decision to continue your gym program (see 'Pregnancy Exercise Guidelines' in Chapter 3).
- Seek individual advice from an exercise consultant during pregnancy.
- As your pregnancy progresses substitute exercises that are specific to pregnancy, such as those given in the Home Exercise Program for Pregnancy in Part 2, for part of your gym routine, and focus on physical preparation for childbirth.
- Make sure your nutrition is adequate to meet the increased energy demands of pregnancy and exercise.
- Consider joining a land- or water-based pregnancy exercise class to meet other women who are changing shape.

I haven't done any regular exercise since leaving school . . .
You are probably a little nervous about not being fit enough to cope with the pregnancy, birth and motherhood, yet you may also be concerned about the safety of exercise for yourself and your baby.

What should you focus on?

▶ Congratulate yourself for deciding to make a start.

▶ Try the Home Exercise Program for Pregnancy given in Part 2: you can be confident that all the exercises in this book are specially designed for pregnant women and new mothers. They are appropriate for you if your pregnancy is healthy. To reassure yourself, discuss your concerns with your medical consultant.

▶ Add a general aerobic activity, such as walking or swimming for 15 to 20 minutes a couple of times per week, and you'll see a marked improvement in your ability to do your normal activities, even though you are getting heavier as your pregnancy progresses.

▶ Work out at a level that is comfortable for you. Initially you may need to take rests between exercises.

▶ Consider joining a specialist pregnancy exercise class so that you can enjoy the company of others and gain reassurance from discussing your needs and concerns with an exercise consultant.

I do aerobics four times per week – more often if I can fit it in . . .
Some might say you are addicted to exercise. You probably enjoy the adrenaline surge from exercise and may find it difficult to reduce your exercise in line with conservative heart-rate guidelines. You may even be inclined to miss your body's signals of exercise stress. You may also find it difficult to accept your body-shape changes and the weight gain associated with a healthy pregnancy. Nevertheless, you are probably concerned about the safety of your exercise choices for your baby.

What should you focus on?

▶ Seek appropriate advice from your medical or exercise consultant.

▶ Remember you do not have to work as hard during pregnancy to achieve the same aerobic benefit from your exercise due to the intrinsic training effect of pregnancy.

▶ Maintain your aerobic level of fitness, but probably change the types of exercise you choose to include more lifestyle activities such as swimming, 'aerobic walking', and using the electronic cardiovascular equipment in the gym. This will vary the stress on your body and hence help prevent injury to your joints and ligaments from repetitive stress. The aerobic-style classes you do should be low impact with minimum choreography, stepping or sliding. You may find it easier to use a pregnancy exercise class as an alternative because then you won't feel the odd one out and you won't have to keep changing exercises.

▶ Allow for rest and recovery within your program so that you meet the metabolic demands of the pregnancy.

▶ Check that you are eating healthily to meet the extra energy and nutritional requirements of your pregnancy. It may be wise to consult a dietician.

▶ Ensure you have adequate hydration to reduce the likelihood of overheating, especially during the first trimester.

▶ Do no more than four aerobic exercise sessions per week, to allow for a rest day between sessions.

▶ Add pregnancy-specific exercise alternatives, especially for your abdominals and thighs, to help prepare you for childbirth: the Home Exercise Program for Pregnancy given in Part 2 will help you choose appropriate exercises.

I have been active all my life and I regularly attended gym and aerobics until I got pregnant . . .

You know the benefits of regular exercise, but the safety of you and your baby is of greater concern to you now than your level of fitness. You need the confidence to start again. First ask yourself why you stopped. Was it because you were unsure of what was safe or because you have been unwell? Obviously you will need to check with your medical consultant before you begin exercising again, but most women who have healthy pregnancies benefit from doing regular pregnancy-specific exercise.

What should you focus on?

▶ Find an exercise class with a supportive atmosphere, where your exercise leader fully understands the needs of pregnancy. It is probably best to consider pregnancy fitness classes and lifestyle aerobic activities — for example, walking, swimming or using cardiovascular exercise equipment such as stationary bikes and treadmills — rather than to go back to general aerobics classes now you've taken a break from exercise.

▶ Perhaps add a light-weights program in the gym to develop endurance in the muscles of your upper back ready for the extra lifting associated with looking after a baby. Talk to an exercise consultant.

▶ Consider joining a pregnancy exercise class to meet other women who are changing shape.

▶ Add the Home Exercise Program given in Part 2 to help you prepare your body physically for pregnancy, childbirth and mothering.

I walk the dog every night after work . . .

Do you walk a big dog 'aerobically' over a long distance or go for a leisurely stroll where your dog stops at every tree?

What should you focus on?

▶ Walk for your aerobic fitness, at a regular pace that makes you feel that you are working 'somewhat to moderately hard' for between 15 to 30 minutes.

▶ Watch the length of your stride, the gradient and the terrain where you walk to protect your pelvic joints from injury.

▶ Add exercises specific to pregnancy, such as the Home Exercise Program for Pregnancy given in Part 2, to help you prepare your body physically for pregnancy, childbirth and mothering.

▶ Consider joining a pregnancy exercise class to meet other women who are changing shape.

I normally play squash/tennis/netball for a local team . . .

You enjoy the competition of sport and the companionship of being in a team. Ask yourself: 'How important is it for me to win? Can I enjoy just a social game?'. Do you think you will know when it's time to stop? Are you looking for an alternative during pregnancy?

What should you focus on?

▶ Congratulate yourself on your initiative to seek alternatives.

▶ Understand the risks associated with continuing your chosen sport: if the sport is highly competitive, it is difficult to notice signals of discomfort. Also check your sport association's rules and insurance. Be aware of the possible risk of injury to yourself and your baby associated with your chosen sport.

▶ Seek advice from your medical or exercise consultant.

▶ Check that your diet is adequate for the energy and nutritional demands of pregnancy and exercise.

▶ When it becomes inappropriate to continue your sport, it is probably best to consider pregnancy fitness classes. Joining a class will help you develop new social contacts with other women who are changing shape.

▶ Remember that activities such as walking and swimming will help you maintain your fitness.

▶ Include exercises specific to pregnancy, such as those given in the Home Exercise Program for Pregnancy in Part 2, to help you prepare your body physically for pregnancy, childbirth and mothering.

I'm busy all day at work and haven't had time for anything regular, although I occasionally walk on weekends . . .

Firstly consider the sort of work you do. Are you a physically active mother at home with another child and without household assistance, or someone in a sedentary occupation, or a woman wearing the hats of both mother and employee? Your normal activity levels will influence the amount and type of physical exercise you need during pregnancy. Importantly, do you consider yourself physically busy or mentally stressed?

What should you focus on?

▶ Congratulate yourself on making time for yourself and your baby — you'll share in the benefits.

▶ Focus on releasing tension and taking time out for yourself.

▶ Enjoy the endorphin effects of exercise — feeling better and sleeping better.

▶ 'Diarise' your exercise time so you get yourself into the habit. Focus on the importance of being physically ready for childbirth so that you do make time for exercise in your schedule. It will take time and practice, but you will appreciate the benefits of more energy during your pregnancy and after childbirth.

▶ Make sure you are eating healthily to meet the nutritional needs of your pregnancy.

▶ Your exercise program should be for aerobic benefit (see Chapter 5), strength and flexibility (see the Home Exercise Program for Pregnancy given in Part 2). A specially designed pregnancy class should offer all of that as well as the discipline of a regular commitment.

I have a long-standing back problem and have treatment regularly, so I can't take part in normal exercise or sport because I have to be very careful . . .

You will probably be very concerned about how your back will stand up to the changes of pregnancy and apprehensive about moving your back at all. You may wonder how your back pain will affect your labour and how you will manage the lifting and carrying of mothering.

What should you focus on?

▶ Seek advice from an exercise consultant and from the physiotherapist or medical consultant treating your condition.

▶ Exercise daily, within your limits, and be alert to the signals to slow down, stop or change your exercise plan.

▶ Consider water exercise: it may be better because you can use the flotation effect of water to relax your back, or swim for aerobic and strength benefits.

▶ Consider walking for the aerobic benefit if your back feels comfortable with this.

▶ Learn to accept your limits of pain so that you can enjoy your mothering experience.

▶ If your consultant is in agreement, strengthen your abdominal, thigh and buttock muscles, using upright, functional exercises that put no strain on your back, such as squats and abdominal bracing. Use pelvic rocking on hands and knees as an exercise to relieve back pain as well as to strengthen your back. You might like to show your consultant the relevant exercises given in the Home Exercise Program for Pregnancy in Part 2.

▶ Seek advice about baby furniture, shelves, trolleys, heights of benches and methods of doing household tasks to minimise stresses on your back.

choosing the right aerobic exercise

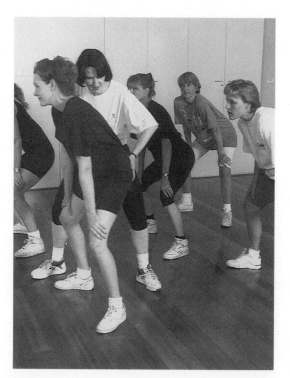

Most recreational pursuits, such as walking and swimming, are aerobic in nature; that is, they have an effect on cardiovascular and respiratory fitness. During this type of exercise, the amount of air taken into the body increases. Working muscles need to be supplied with oxygen. This is usually achieved by a combination of increasing the amount of blood the heart pushes out with each beat (stroke volume) and increasing the frequency with which that blood is pumped out by the heart (heart rate). The heart must pump more blood to working muscles during exercise via the arteries. This increased work is reflected as an increased pulse.

When you exercise you gain a measure of how hard you are working by taking your pulse rate. If you wish to improve the fitness of your cardio-vascular and respiratory systems (that is, achieve aerobic fitness), you need to work within your heart-rate training zone. For the average person, this is usually estimated as working at between 60 and 75 per cent of his or her age-related maximum heart rate. The formula usually used to calculate an individual's maximum heart rate is 220 minus age. For example, a woman who is 30 years old has an estimated maximum heart rate of 220 minus 30; that is, 190 beats per minute. If she wishes to train in an aerobic zone of 60 to 75 per cent of her maximum heart rate, her pulse rate should range between 60 per cent of 190 (that is, 114 beats per minute) and 75 per cent of 190 (that is, 142 beats per minute).

As outlined in the 'Pregnancy Exercise Guidelines' in Chapter 3, aerobic work in pregnancy should be at a level perceived to be 'somewhat to moderately hard', and in a range of between 60 and 75 per cent of your maximum heart rate, with a suggested upper limit of 140 beats per minute, for a duration consistent with previous experience and exercise intensity. This is a general guide, which you can discuss with your medical or exercise consultant.

Some recreational pursuits are more suitable for pregnancy than others. If you have previously participated in a particular sport or aerobic activity you may, with advice, be able to continue it at a modified level during pregnancy. The following information is written mainly for women who have enjoyed these types of exercise regularly or are looking to start an exercise program now they are pregnant. If you have exercised at a competitive level before your pregnancy, you should read the following for general advice and then discuss the suitability of continuing your previous activity with your medical or exercise consultant.

WALKING

The benefits of walking are:

▶ it can be done at any time
▶ it is a pleasant way of spending time with your partner or friends
▶ it can be easily altered to fit the pregnancy exercise guidelines
▶ it does not cost anything, except for the purchase of a supportive and well-cushioned pair of shoes.

ADVICE

▶ Avoid walking on concrete where there are softer alternatives.

▶ Avoid rugged bush-walking, soft sand and steep gradients because walking on uneven terrain may cause pelvic-joint and back pain.

▶ Wear your well-fitting exercise shoes every time you walk.

▶ Walk tall with good posture.

▶ Hug your baby with your abdominal muscles and brace your pelvic-floor muscles as you walk.

▶ Swing your arms freely with slightly bent elbows to assist your walking and relaxation.

▶ If you feel any back or pelvic pain, shorten the length of your stride slightly, check your pelvic tuck and slow down a little.

▶ Avoid power walking, where your heel impact and stride length may cause discomfort.

Walking Plan

▶ Warm up by walking at a slow to moderate pace for 5 minutes, then stretch your calf and thigh muscles.

▶ Increase your pace until you feel you are working moderately hard and continue at this pace for 15 minutes.

▶ Cool down by slowing to a stroll for 5 minutes.

▶ Finish with stretches of your calf and thigh muscles and pelvic rocking (see Exercise 3 in the Home Exercise Program for Pregnancy given in Part 2).

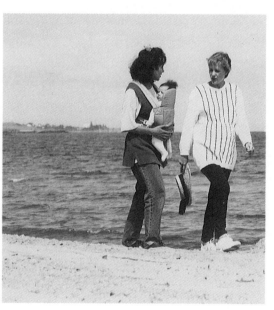

▶ As your fitness increases, gradually build up the aerobic part of your walk until you are walking for a total of 30 minutes.

▶ Don't forget your water bottle, and choose a cool time for your walk.

SWIMMING

The benefits of swimming are:

▶ it relieves stress on your lower limb joints, due to the flotation effect of the water, so it feels good
▶ it is excellent aerobic exercise
▶ the intensity can be altered to suit your energy levels at the time
▶ your strokes can be altered to vary the muscles you use
▶ standing and walking in waist-deep water may help reduce the swelling of your legs in late pregnancy.

ADVICE

▶ Swim in water less than 30°C as you can overheat without realising it.
▶ Limit your effort to 'somewhat to moderately hard' as you can become fatigued quicker in water than on land.
▶ Avoid breast-stroke kick and butterfly stroke because of the stresses these place on your back and pelvic joints.
▶ Cool down well before you leave the pool by walking in the shallow end of the pool or by relaxed floating, as your blood pressure can drop suddenly when you get out of the water.
▶ Be sure to add backstroke to your swimming routine in order to vary the stresses on your back.

Swimming Plan

▶ Warm up by swimming in the slow lane for 5 minutes, then stretch your arms, back and legs before you begin your vigorous swimming.
▶ Increase your pace until you are swimming at a 'somewhat to moderately hard' pace and maintain this for 15 minutes. (If you are not a regular swimmer, gradually build up to this amount.)
▶ Cool down by swimming in the slow lane for 5 minutes, then walking in the shallow end or floating for relaxation.
▶ If you feel any discomfort around your pelvis during or after swimming, consider swimming with a pool buoy between your legs or seek advice from an exercise consultant.

Remember Do not swim or exercise in hydrotherapy pools, or relax in hot spas or baths, because the water temperature of these is usually greater than 30°C.

STATIONARY BIKE RIDING

The benefits of stationary bike riding are:

- it combines aerobic exercise with leg strengthening (which is needed for sustaining labour positions and for safe lifting)
- it can be done at your own convenience and combined with other leisure activities, such as reading, talking or watching television
- the resistance on the bike can be altered to vary the emphasis of your exercise from aerobic work (light resistance) to developing strength (heavier resistance).

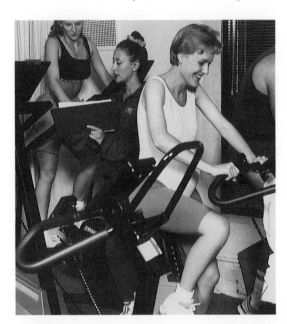

Riding a stationary bike gives an aerobic benefit without the risk of falling.

ADVICE

- The bike seat should be wide enough to be comfortable and may need to be tilted slightly forward.
- In late pregnancy, you may need to sit on a small cushion or folded towel.
- Raise the seat to a height that requires your legs to almost straighten as you pedal, and sit up tall.
- In late pregnancy, there is a possibility of groin pressure and leg swelling if you bike ride for long periods of time without a break.
- While recumbent bikes are considered by some to have advantages for pregnancy, be guided by comfort. Potentially these bikes may decrease the blood flow in your legs as the weight of your baby increases.
- Occasionally do some full-range arm movements to increase the blood flow in your arms.
- To gain maximum aerobic benefits, maintain the bike resistance between light and moderate, and cycle comfortably for up to 15 minutes. Heavy resistance increases the risk of pelvic-joint pain.

LOW-IMPACT AEROBICS

The benefits of low-impact aerobics are:

▶ if you are experienced and follow the advice below, aerobics classes can be a good total work-out, combining the aerobic, strength and flexibility components of fitness

▶ there are many styles of aerobics classes, so there's probably one to suit you – a pregnancy-specific aerobics class will give you a great all-round work-out while taking into account your special needs.

CAUTIONS

▶ Unless you are experienced at this form of exercise, aerobics classes may not be suitable because of the speed of the music, the type of choreography and the length of the aerobic section within the class.

▶ The very thing that makes aerobics classes fun – the movement and energy of the group – may cause you to forget the safety factors for pregnancy exercise.

ADVICE

▶ Look for low-impact and lightly choreographed classes to lessen the risk of injury and overheating.

▶ Limit your step width and step length to protect your pelvic joints from injury.

▶ Control your steps during fast choreography – do not feel you have to keep up with the class.

▶ Limit your changes of direction to no more than 90-degree turns, unless you step the turn around.

▶ Do not do any high-impact moves, bouncing or propulsions. Change the move to a low-impact option.

▶ Keep your knees 'soft' to protect your knees, back and pelvic joints.

▶ Brace your abdominal and pelvic-floor muscles, and maintain good posture throughout the class.

▶ Change the abdominal exercises in the floor section of the class to those suitable for pregnancy (see the Home Exercise Program for Pregnancy given in Part 2).

▶ Avoid step- and slide-class styles to reduce the risk of pelvic-joint pain.

Of course the best low-impact aerobic exercise class is one specially designed for pregnancy, where you can relax and enjoy your exercise because you know that the class has been designed to be safe for you and your baby.

GYM PROGRAM

The benefits of a gym program are:

▶ it is specifically designed for you
▶ by combining cardiovascular equipment with light weights, it can give you a total work-out, covering all components of fitness
▶ it can be done in your own time and at your own pace
▶ it can be supervised, monitored and adjusted throughout your pregnancy.

Individual advice from an exercise consultant will help you design the program that is right for you and your baby.

Some gym equipment is specifically designed for aerobic exercise. Use the treadmill, steppers, bikes and other equipment for their aerobic benefits, remembering to use a low resistance to avoid pelvic-joint stresses and raising your blood pressure.

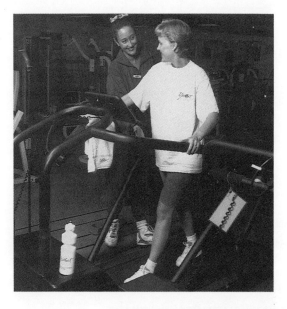

ADVICE REGARDING CARDIOVASCULAR EQUIPMENT

▶ Apply the advice for walking and stationary bike riding.
▶ For the best aerobic benefits, exercise for an equal length of time on each machine, stopping at the point where you feel you could still do more. Build up to a combined aerobic routine lasting about 20 minutes.
▶ Avoid any equipment that causes discomfort during or after your exercise, especially in your pelvis or back.

ADVICE REGARDING LIGHT WEIGHTS

▶ Reduce your weights by approximately 20 to 25 per cent, so that you can do ten to fifteen repetitions while you maintain good posture. Adjust your weights regularly as your pregnancy progresses.

- Aim for endurance (lower resistance, higher repetitions) rather than strength gains (higher resistance, lower repetitions) in your work-out.
- Alternate arm and leg exercises within your routine to avoid blood pooling and blood pressure changes.
- Don't do prolonged work with overhead weights because of the risk of increasing your heart rate and blood pressure.
- Breathe out as you push against the weight.
- Avoid free weights where there is a danger of them dropping on your abdomen.
- As your pregnancy progresses, consider changing to hydraulic equipment, rather than pin-loaded, if you are having difficulty controlling the return, or eccentric, phase of your exercises.

STEP, SLIDE, CIRCUIT AND BOX-A-CISE CLASSES

Even though many consider step, slide, circuit and box-a-cise routines are good forms of aerobic exercise during the first trimester for women experienced at doing these classes, the risks appear to outweigh the benefits. We at Changing Shape believe aerobic benefits can be better achieved by other forms of exercise without risk to your back and pelvic joints or danger of overheating and falling.

CAUTIONS FOR STEP CLASSES

- Repetitive asymmetrical or unilateral movements and step choreography can cause uneven pressure on your pelvic joints and lead to instability in those joints.
- The motivational effect of the music and group movement can be a risk because you can go past the safety stage.
- There is an increased risk of tripping or falling when stepping, especially in a crowded or a highly choreographed class.

ADVICE FOR STEP CLASSES

- If you feel you must step, decrease the height of the step, or use the platform only.
- Reduce the length of time you spend stepping up and down within the class. Try replacing some exercises with floor-based alternatives.
- Make sure you drink enough to maintain your hydration in these classes.

CAUTION FOR SLIDE CLASSES

The constant sideways movements may strain the groin or aggravate pelvic-joint instability.

ADVICE FOR SLIDE CLASSES

Slide movements are not functional unless you ski as a routine part of your everyday life and are therefore not recommended in pregnancy.

CAUTION FOR CIRCUIT CLASSES

While the concept of circuit classes is excellent for an all-round work-out, the speed of the music and the need to keep up with the pace of the group may be risky during pregnancy.

ADVICE FOR CIRCUIT CLASSES

Be prepared to reduce the speed at which you work and avoid some stations.

CAUTION FOR BOX-A-CISE CLASSES

The sustained upper-body work can be a risk factor for increasing blood pressure and heart rate and is therefore not recommended in pregnancy.

Enjoy discussing your plans with friends who understand what it's like to change shape.

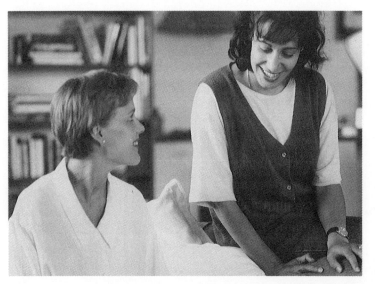

While all these classes are popular at present, new styles of exercise are constantly being evolved. Examine each new fad on its own merits and for its relevance to pregnancy. For pregnancy, exercise programs should be functional, supervised and previously participated in. Otherwise choose a specifically designed pregnancy exercise class, where new participants can feel comfortable and safe in an environment with other pregnant women. It makes sense to exercise in varied ways during pregnancy (cross-training), to reduce repetitive stresses on your softened joints. So, choose swimming, walking or another aerobic activity, join a pregnancy-specific exercise class and do the Home Exercise Program for Pregnancy given in Part 2 for a complete work-out. For both your and your baby's optimal health, work out aerobically three or four times per week on alternate days. Add your pregnancy-specific exercise at least three times per week. And remember, *rest and recovery* are very important in pregnancy for your baby's growth and development. Above all, LISTEN TO YOUR BODY.

The next part of the book includes the Home Exercise Program for Pregnancy, then in Part 3 you'll find a discussion of exercise alternatives for the early months of motherhood, and the Home Exercise Program for After Childbirth. You can start the latter program shortly after your baby is born. Both home exercise programs have been designed so that you can work through them efficiently. Tips and variations have been included to highlight certain points and to allow you to develop a program that suits your needs.

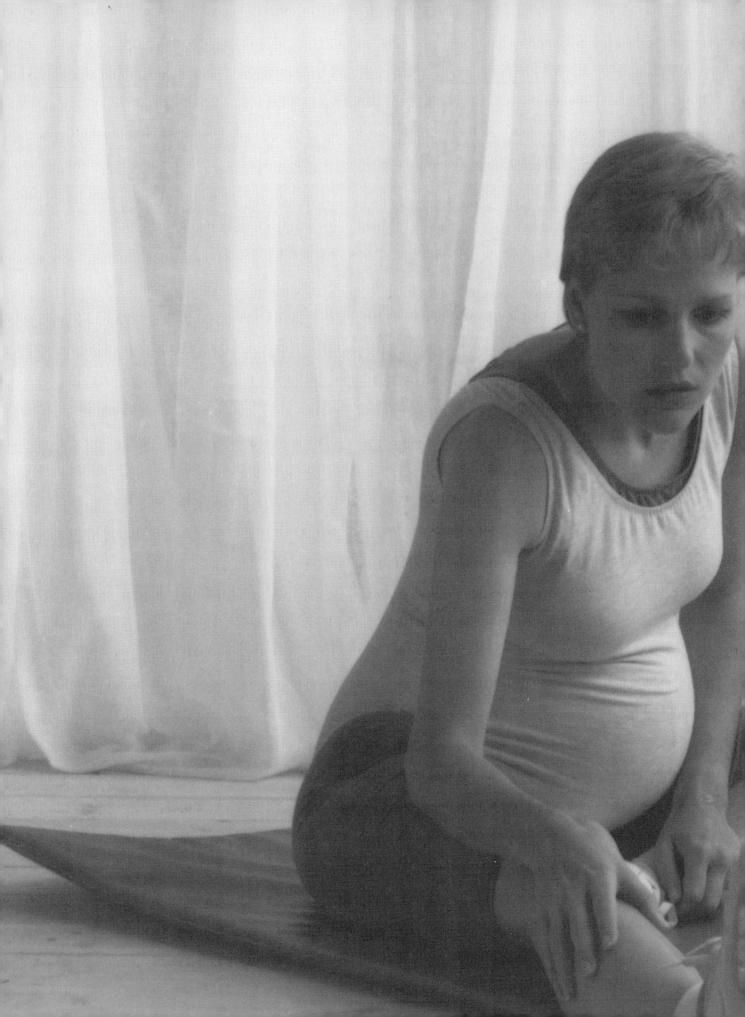

home exercise program for pregnancy

beginning the exercises

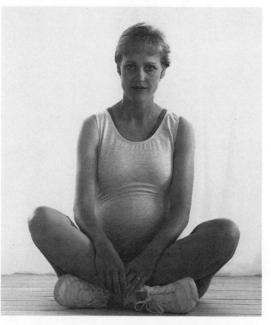

The Home Exercise Program for Pregnancy is designed for you to do at home during your pregnancy. Please note that, while the exercises have been specifically designed for pregnancy, you should consult your medical or exercise consultant for personal advice. Obviously the earlier in pregnancy you start this exercise program, the better your strength and flexibility will be, both during that time and after the birth. But if you're starting later in pregnancy, you will still gain significant benefit.

As we discussed in Part I, the ideal exercise program in pregnancy is one that takes into account both you and your unborn child and is adjusted as your pregnancy progresses. It should balance the major components of fitness — stamina (aerobic fitness), strength and flexibility — with specific exercises designed to allow you to cope with pregnancy more comfortably and prepare your body for childbirth and motherhood.

Choose aerobic activities that appeal to you and are within your level of ability from those discussed in Chapter 5, and do these three to four times per week. You should allow a rest day between sessions to reduce the potential risk of over-exercise. The Home Exercise Program for strength and flexibility should complement your chosen aerobic activities. You should aim to do it at least three times per week, but it can be done daily.

Your exercise should be enjoyable. If you find you are uncomfortable or fatigued or feel you are pushing yourself, your choice of exercise is probably not right for you at the moment. Consider changing your program, reducing the number of times you are exercising or adjusting the amount of time you spend exercising each session.

For best results, balance your exercise with adequate rest to allow your body to cope with the extra metabolic work of pregnancy. Remember, as your pregnancy progresses you will probably find you cannot do as much physical work. This is quite normal as your body is getting heavier as your baby grows, and the increasing weight is adding to your body's workload. If your body is rested, as well as appropriately fit, you usually feel better during pregnancy and are able to recover quicker physically after the birth.

FOLLOWING THE HOME EXERCISE PROGRAM

The Home Exercise Program for Pregnancy follows through logically from one position to the next, rather than organising exercises by body region or muscle groups worked. This allows your exercise to be efficient — both in terms of time spent and of avoiding potential stress on your body structures.

The exercises are ordered so that you warm up, stabilise, work and stretch in each position before you have to change position. For best results you should follow the order of exercises suggested for each position. Exercises 1 to 12 are done in an upright position; Exercises 13 to 17 are done on hands and knees; Exercises 18 to 21 are done in a lying position; and Exercises 22 to 26 are done in the sitting position. Depending on your comfort and the time available, you can choose either to finish your program with relaxation in the sitting position or move onto your side. Tips, variations and cautions have been included to allow you to adjust your program to suit your body and pregnancy.

While you will probably find the exercise names and photos are a sufficient cue as you become more familiar with the program, reread the copy from time to time to remind yourself about correct technique so that you reduce the risk of discomfort.

The number of times you do each exercise at a time is called the number of repetitions. After a short rest, you may wish to repeat the exercise. This is known as doing a second set. For example, two sets of six repetitions means you did the exercise six times, took a short rest and then did six repetitions a second time.

Usually the number of repetitions suggested in the text for each exercise is eight. If you feel you are unable to achieve the number recommended, do what you feel comfortable with. As your fitness develops you may feel able to do more. As your pregnancy progresses you may need to do fewer. If an exercise does not feel right, leave it out of your program and discuss it with your medical or exercise consultant. Depending on the number of repetitions you do, the program may last for 20 minutes.

We have recommended holding a comfortable stretch for a minimum of 10 seconds in the case of most stretches. However, only hold the stretch while it feels comfortable, to help prevent injury from muscle and soft tissue tightness. To develop your flexibility you may like gradually to increase the length of time you hold the feeling of a comfortable stretch up to 30 seconds, and perhaps repeat the stretch after a short rest. Remember, after you have held a stretch, to return to your starting position slowly to help prevent strain.

You will not need to purchase any expensive equipment to do the Home Exercise Program for Pregnancy, but you will need to consider the environment in which you plan to exercise. Don't do the floor-exercise section of the program on a bed as it will not give your body adequate support, but you can substitute a rest on a bed for the relaxation section.

When planning your exercise session, you should consider the following points.

▶ Allow time for these exercises. Don't stop abruptly. Getting up suddenly may be the cause of injury, so don't answer the phone or door or have anything cooking while you exercise.

▶ If it is a hot day, exercise in an air-conditioned area or early in the morning or in the evening, and make sure there is a good air-flow around you.

- Wear supportive footwear and loose, comfortable clothes, with no tight elastic bands around the waist or legs.
- Exercise on a clear, non-slip floor surface to avoid accidents.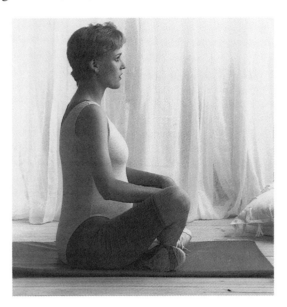
- Drink water regularly while you exercise to avoid dehydration.
- Breathe evenly and easily during your exercises.
- To protect your joints, change positions slowly and smoothly, keeping your knees together as your move.
- Never overstrain yourself: allow *no* pain. Always work within your comfort zone.
- Brace your pelvic-floor and abdominal muscles during all exercises (see Chapter 2).
- Be aware of keeping a balanced posture during all exercises. Move smoothly and at a steady pace throughout your exercise.
- Add music for your pleasure and motivation. Choose music that has a walking-pace beat. You may like to count your repetitions in eights to the beat of the music.

Check that your posture is balanced and your abdominal muscles are braced during all exercise to protect your back from strain.

You can vary the program according to your needs by:

- reducing the time spent on each position by reducing the number of repetitions
- choosing to do only one position each session
- increasing the number of sets of repetitions
- repeating all the exercises of one position before moving on to the next.

Now – let's get started!

the program

Each time you begin: LISTEN TO YOUR BODY.

▶ *Is it right for you today?*

▶ *Be prepared to stop exercising if you have any unusual feelings or pain.*

▶ *If any exercise doesn't feel quite right or causes discomfort, leave it out.*

▶ *Discuss any changes you make with your medical or exercise consultant.*

WARM-UP

Why warm up? When you begin to exercise, your warm-up will prepare your body for exercise by:

▶ increasing the blood flow to your muscles
▶ giving you a feel for movement, and therefore
▶ reducing the risk of injury to your body from exercise.

Because the exercises in this program are designed to flow from one to the next, you are warming up your body as you move through the early part of the program. Adding a 5-minute easy walk or being generally active before starting the program should ensure your body is ready for exercise.

1

JOGGING ON THE SPOT

This exercise is not essential if you have just returned from a walk.

▶ Hold your pelvis tucked in and 'press-stud', or brace, your abdominal muscles (see Chapter 2).

▶ Brace your pelvic-floor muscles (see Chapter 2).

▶ Jog, keeping your toes on the floor.

▶ Let your arms swing freely as you jog.

▶ Jog until you feel warm.

VARIATIONS

1 Jog as described above, but punch in front of you with your fists at chest height.
2 Alternate arm movements – move from eight biceps curls, bending your elbows beside your body, to eight forward punches.

Remember to keep your feet moving between sets of exercises to prevent blood pooling in your legs.

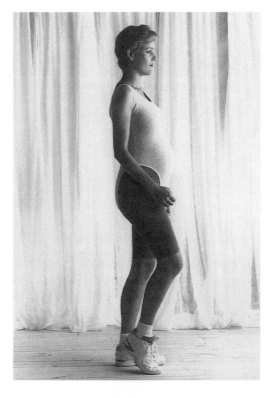

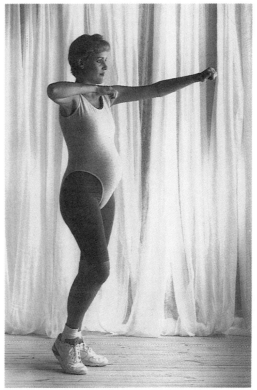

Top Jogging on the spot.
Bottom Variation 1.

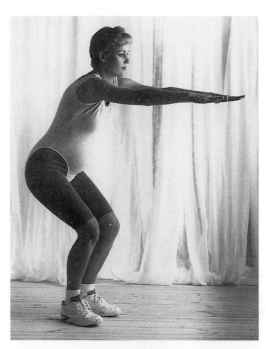

2

SIT-BACKS

- Stand with your feet a comfortable distance apart and parallel.

- Keep your weight on your heels.

- Tuck in your pelvis to prevent your back arching, and keep your pelvic floor braced.

- Let your knees bend and 'sit' back as if you were going to sit on a high stool.

- Swing your arms forward for balance.

- Rise up, pushing your arms back.

- Repeat in sets of eight.

- Alternate this exercise with jogging on the spot (Exercise 1).

TIPS TO PREVENT KNEE PAIN

- Your knees should stay pointing in line with your toes.
- As you sit back, watch that your knees are not further forward than your toes.

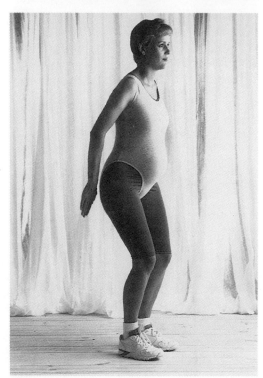

3

PELVIC ROCKING OR BELLY DANCING

Starting position

▶ Stand tall, with your legs apart, just wider than your shoulders, and with your toes turned out slightly.

▶ Relax your shoulders and rest your hands on your hips or under your tummy.

▶ Keep your knees in line with your toes.

▶ Bend your knees until you are just above bar-stool height.

▶ Brace your pelvic floor.

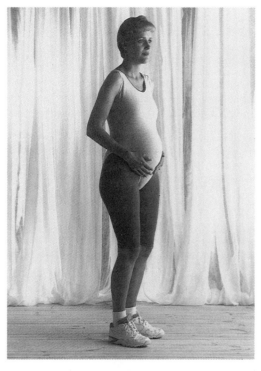

Exercise

▶ Tuck your tail under and hug your baby towards your spine, using your abdominal muscles.

▶ Release.

▶ Repeat the exercise in sets of eight, then return to your normal tall standing posture.

VARIATION

Some women find this a difficult exercise to learn while standing. You may find it easier to begin in the hands and knees position given for pelvic rocking (Exercise 14), progress to leaning forward onto a bench, and then go into this position.

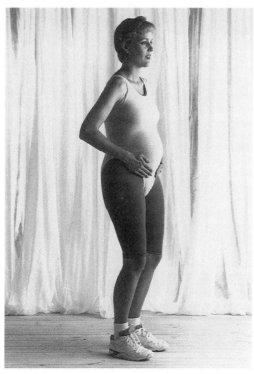

PELVIC ROCKING OR BELLY DANCING *continued*

TIP FOR POSTURE

To ensure your back is straight and tall, visualise:

▶ a rod across your shoulders
▶ a book balancing on your head.

SIDE PELVIC LIFTS

▶ Position yourself as for pelvic rocking (see the top photograph for Exercise 3).

▶ Hug your baby to your spine.

▶ Hitch up your pelvis and rock gently from side to side.

▶ Repeat the exercise eight times, alternating sides: both sides count as one repetition.

VARIATIONS

1 Alternate side pelvic lifts with pelvic rocking (Exercise 3) so that the movement is similar to belly dancing; that is, lift one side, pelvic rock, lift the other side, pelvic rock . . . You can do this with your feet close together or apart.

2 With your feet together or apart, draw imaginary circles with your pelvis in both directions, as in belly dancing.

5
ANKLE EXERCISES

‣ Stand tall, with your feet wider than your shoulders, and your hands resting on your hips.

‣ Maintain your pelvic tuck (hug your baby) and keep your pelvic floor braced.

‣ Raise your right then your left heel without rocking your body sideways.

‣ Raise your right then your left toes without rocking your body sideways.

‣ Repeat the exercise in sets of eight heel lifts, followed by eight toe raises.

VARIATION

Add alternating biceps curls, bending your elbows beside your body, as you lift your heel or toes.

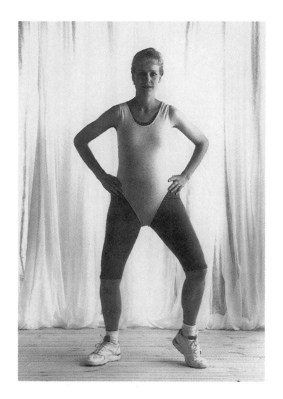

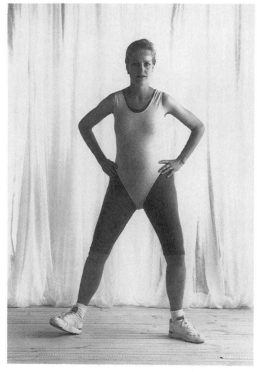

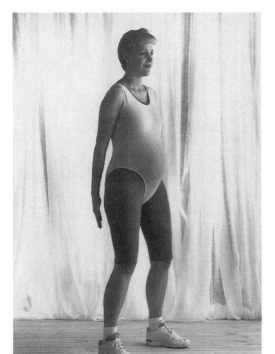

6

HANDS IN BACK POCKETS

Starting position

▶ Stand tall, with your feet wider apart than your shoulders, and let your hands rest behind your bottom.

▶ Bend your knees slightly. .

▶ Maintain your pelvic tuck and brace your pelvic floor.

Exercise

▶ Place your hands as if in your back pockets.

▶ Raise your elbows (keeping them pointing backwards), then lower them.

▶ Repeat the exercise in sets of eight.

VARIATIONS

The following are harder options.

1 Bring your hands closer together before you lift your elbows.
2 Combine the exercise with squats (Exercise 7), lifting your elbows up as you raise your body to a standing position.

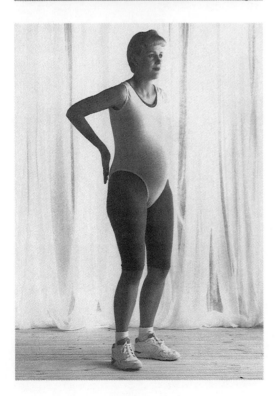

7

PLIES OR SQUATS

Starting position

▶ Stand tall, with your feet wider apart than your shoulders and your hands on your hips, your shoulders relaxed and your eyes looking ahead.

▶ Bend your knees slightly.

▶ Let your weight come back on your heels.

▶ Maintain your pelvic tuck and keep your pelvic floor braced.

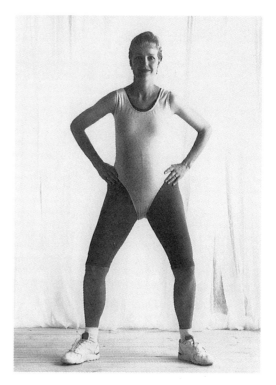

Exercise

▶ Bend your knees as if you were sliding down an imaginary wall, until you are slightly lower than bar-stool height.

▶ Keep your knees in line with your toes by turning out from your hips.

▶ Rise up to your full height, pulling up through your thighs.

▶ Repeat the exercise, building up to sets of eight.

POSTURE CHECK TO HELP AVOID KNEE PAIN

Is your weight on your heels and the outside borders of your feet, and can you wriggle your toes?

VARIATION

You may like to combine the exercise with the hands in back pockets exercise (Exercise 6), or chest presses (Exercise 8), or both, when you are stronger.

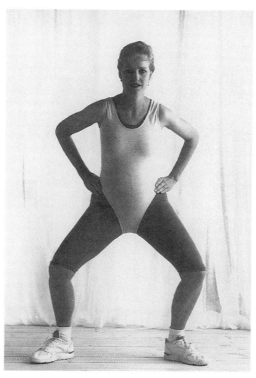

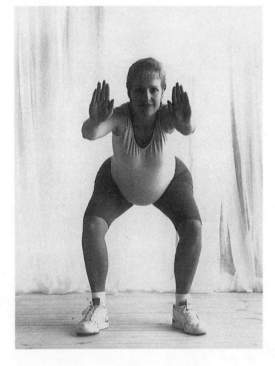

 8

CHEST PRESSES

◗ Stand tall, with your feet wider apart than your shoulders and your hands at about shoulder height.

◗ Maintain your pelvic tuck.

◗ Stretch your arms forward, with your elbows level with your shoulders.

◗ Then pull your arms back smoothly and firmly, bringing your hands level with your chest so that your elbows are behind your shoulders.

◗ Repeat the exercise in sets of eight.

VARIATION

A harder option is to combine the exercise with squats, as shown in the second photograph.

ADJUSTMENT

If you experience any back pain or discomfort during this exercise:

◗ do not combine it with a squat (do it in the upright standing position)
◗ check that you are maintaining your pelvic tuck
◗ bring your hands down from chest height towards waist level.

Top Chest presses.
Bottom Variation.

9

PELVIC-FLOOR EXERCISES

See Chapter 2 for a detailed explanation.

▶ Stand in the starting position for squats (see the top photograph for Exercise 7).

▶ Squeeze your pelvic-floor muscles, lifting up inside.

▶ Hold, then release.

▶ Repeat the exercise in sets of eight.

Note It is a good idea to repeat this exercise in the hands and knees, side-lying and sitting positions.

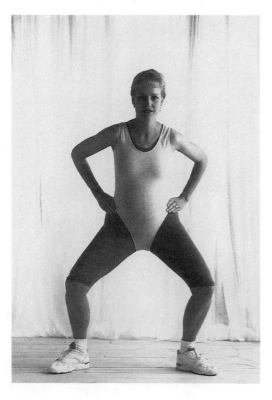

10

DEEP SQUATS

- Stand in the starting position for squats (see the first photograph for Exercise 7).

- Lean your body slightly forward from your hips.

- Sit back into a deep squat (aiming to be about chair-seat height). Let your hands slide forward along your upper legs towards your knees (see the photograph opposite).

- Rise up to bar-stool height.

- Repeat the exercise, building up to sets of eight.

CAUTIONS

- It is essential to check your knee posture very carefully (see Exercise 2), and to keep your abdominals braced to help prevent back pain.
- Make sure you shake your legs or move your feet between sets to avoid knee pain and blood pooling.
- Limit the number of times you go up and down because too many squats may aggravate knee pain.

VARIATIONS

1   To work harder: gradually increase the time you hold the squat before rising.
2   You can do your pelvic rocking (Exercise 3) in the deep squat position.
3   To test your strength and flexibility, squat down as if to sit on a low stool, hold the position, then rise to chair-seat height. Limit your number of repetitions to sets of four.

TIP FOR LABOUR

Spending time sitting on a low stool in a squatting position with your knees turned out will improve your hip flexibility for upright birthing positions. Watch the television or read the newspaper in this position.

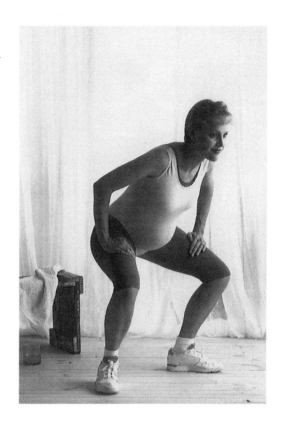

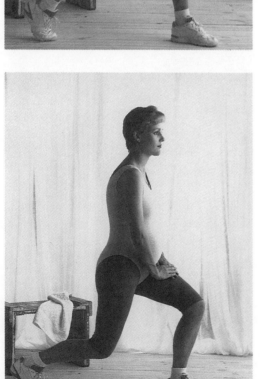

11

DIPS

▶ Stand tall, then take one step back and place your weight on that leg, with your heel raised.

▶ Continue to stand tall, keeping your shoulders, hips and back knee in a straight line.

▶ Maintain your pelvic tuck and keep your pelvic floor braced throughout the exercise.

▶ Lower your back knee towards the floor without lunging forward over your front knee.

▶ Rise to the starting position.

▶ Repeat the exercise, building up to sets of eight.

▶ Repeat with the other leg.

CAUTION

If this exercise causes pain or discomfort around your pelvis, leave it out until you feel stronger. If the pain or discomfort continues, you should seek advice from your exercise consultant.

TIP FOR POSTURE

To keep your back straight and prevent your front knee coming forward past your toes, visualise a rod across your shoulders or balancing a book on your head.

12
CALF STRETCHES

Do both these exercises.

Exercise A

▶ Stand tall, then take one step back and place your weight on that leg.

▶ Place your hands on your front thigh.

▶ Look forward, keeping your back straight and long.

▶ Keep your back heel pressed down, with the toes pointing forward.

▶ Lean forward, bending your front knee until you feel a stretch in the back calf muscle.

▶ Hold the position for at least 10 seconds.

▶ Repeat the exercise, using your other leg.

Exercise B

▶ Take a step to bring your back leg in towards your front leg.

▶ Keep your weight on your back leg, your hands on your front thigh and your back straight and long.

▶ Lower your body by bending your knees, until you feel a stretch in your back calf muscle.

▶ Hold the position for at least 10 seconds.

▶ Repeat the exercise, using your other leg.

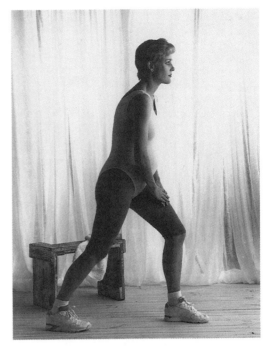

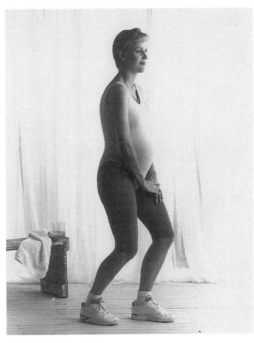

Top Exercise A.
Bottom Exercise B.

CALF STRETCHES *continued*

TIPS

▸ Stretch your calf muscles after walking to help reduce the risk of calf cramps.

▸ Do stretches to improve your flexibility and help you achieve deep squats more comfortably.

TRANSFERRING TO THE HANDS AND KNEES POSITION

▸ Stand with your feet shoulder-width apart.

▸ Bend your knees, sliding your hands down your thighs as you do so.

▸ Place your hands on the floor and take your weight on them.

▸ Let your knees come down to the floor.

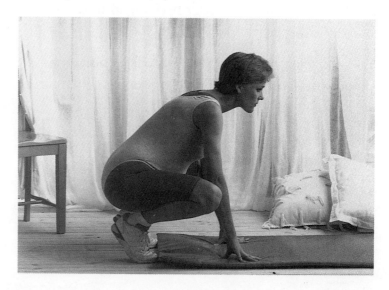

13
CAT STRETCHES

- From the hands and knees position, bring your knuckles close to your knees.

- 'Press-stud', or brace, your abdominals.

- Round your back to hug your baby towards your spine.

- Curl your head under to look to the floor and tuck your tail under.

- Hold the position for a moment to feel the stretch.

- Release your back and return to the neutral position.

- Lift your eyes until they are gazing ahead.

- Hold the position for a moment to feel the stretch.

- Return to the neutral position.

- Repeat the exercise slowly in sets of eight.

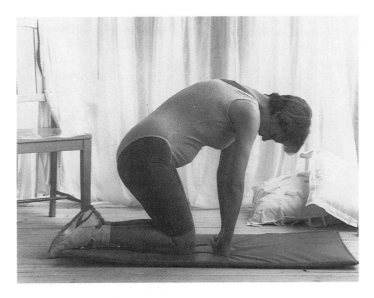

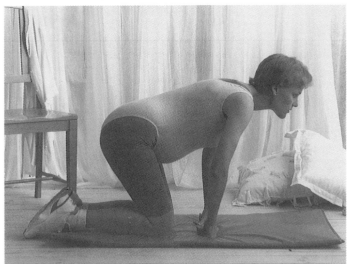

14

PELVIC ROCKING

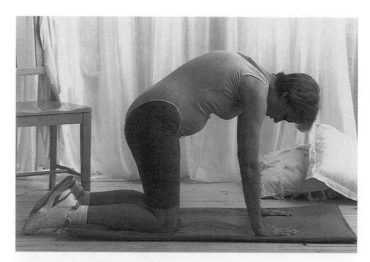

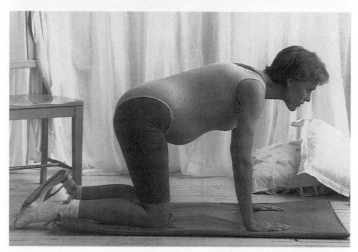

- ▶ In the hands and knees position, let your elbows bend slightly, keeping your hands in line with your shoulders.

- ▶ Take your weight evenly on your hands and knees.

- ▶ 'Press-stud', or brace, your abdominals and maintain this throughout the exercise.

- ▶ Round your back and lift your baby towards your spine, focusing on your breath out as you lift.

- ▶ Release to return to neutral, breathing in as you do so.

- ▶ Repeat the exercise in sets of eight.

ADJUSTMENT

If you experience any wrist pain, you may prefer to take the weight on your knuckles rather than your wrists.

TIP FOR BACK AND PELVIC-JOINT PAIN

Doing pelvic rocking frequently during the day, in this and other positions, will help to relieve the pressure on your back and pelvic joints. It also develops strength in your abdominal muscles, which will help support your back.

15
PUSH-UPS

The emphasis during this exercise is on maintaining a straight back while you raise and lower your shoulders. It is therefore better to focus on keeping your abdominals braced and your back straight, rather than on lowering yourself all the way to the floor.

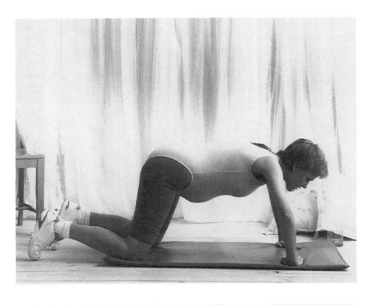

▶ In the hands and knees position, keep your knees comfortably together in line with your hips, and your hands in line with your shoulders.

▶ Keep your back straight by 'press-studding', or bracing, your abdominal muscles.

▶ Bend your elbows and lower your shoulders slowly towards the floor, breathing in as you do so.

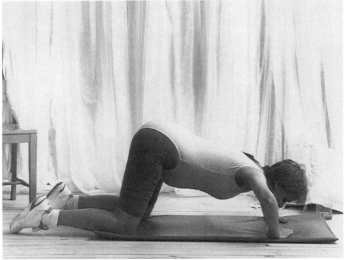

▶ Push yourself up, letting your breath out as you rise.

▶ Repeat the exercise, building up to sets of eight.

ADJUSTMENT

For comfort change your hands position to any of these:

▶ wider apart
▶ closer together
▶ fingers pointed forward or inward.

PUSH-UPS *continued*

VARIATION

To increase the difficulty of the exercise: bring your arms further forward, lean your weight on your hands, cross your ankles and lift your feet off the floor.

16

SPINAL ROTATION

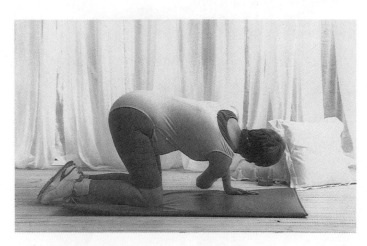

- In the hands and knees position, distribute your weight evenly between one hand and both your knees.

- Bend the elbow of your supporting arm slightly.

- Maintain your pelvic tuck.

- Bring your other arm through smoothly under your body.

- Look under to that side.

- Bring your arm up and back, and turn your head to look towards your elbow.

- Repeat the rotation four times on one side, then change arms.

17

STRETCH-BACKS

- In the hands and knees position, rest on your elbows, with your knees apart but toes together.

- Sit back towards your heels until you feel a stretch in your lower back or buttocks.

- Walk your fingers forward, lowering your chest as you do so, to give a comfortable stretch to your spine.

- Hold the position for as long as you feel comfortable.

- Return to resting on your elbows.

- Repeat the exercise.

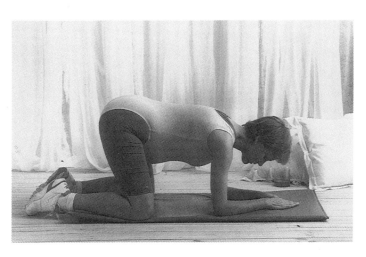

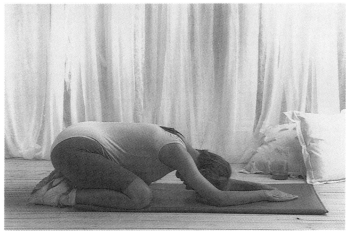

CAUTIONS

- The longer you hold this stretch, the more careful you will need to be when changing position afterwards. Bring your knees together and repeat the pelvic rocking (Exercise 14) before continuing with your program.
- If your knees hurt or the position aggravates heartburn or haemorrhoids, do *not* do this stretch.
- If you feel any pelvic-joint pain during this stretch, alter your position to that for Variation I (see next page).

STRETCH-BACKS *continued*

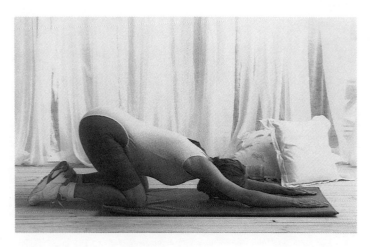

VARIATIONS

1   To add an upper-body stretch, lift your buttocks off your heels while your arms are stretched forward and your chest is close to the floor.

2   While all the weight of your baby is off your pelvic floor as you rest in the elbows and knees position, do some pelvic-floor exercises.

TIP TO RELIEVE SCIATIC PAIN

This can be an excellent stretch to relieve sciatic pain. How far you sit back towards your heels may be limited by pain. Sit back gently to the point where you just begin to feel pain. Hold still until it eases.

TRANSFERRING TO LYING ON YOUR SIDE

▶ In the hands and knees position, bring your knees together.

▶ Hug your baby with your abdominals.

▶ Gently roll your hips to one side and lower yourself, via your elbows, to the floor.

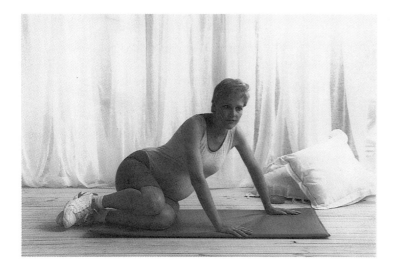

Do Exercises 18 to 21 on one side, before changing to your other side to repeat the exercises.

18
SIDE-LYING PELVIC ROCKING

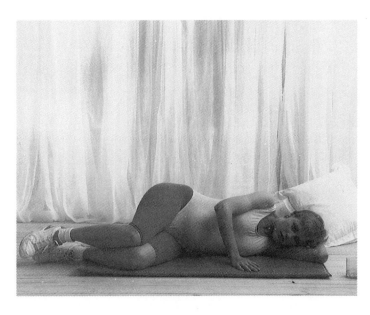

- Lying on your side, bring your knees forward, with one resting on top of the other.

- 'Press-stud', or brace, your abdominals.

- Rock your pelvis back, hugging your baby with your abdominals.

- Breathe out as you rock.

- Release your pelvis, breathing in as you do so.

- Repeat the exercise in sets of eight.

TIP FOR SLEEPING

Lying on your side can be a good sleeping position with or without a pillow between your knees. It may help to reduce the discomfort sometimes experienced in your lower back and pelvic joints.

As your pregnancy progresses, or if you have a separation of your tummy muscles, it may be better to leave Exercises 19 and 20 out of your program. Discuss your individual needs with your exercise consultant.

19

SIDE ABDOMINAL LIFTS

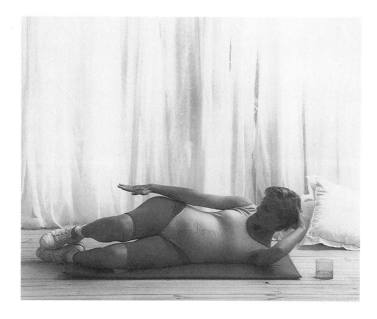

▶ Lie on your side, with your head resting on your lower hand and your top arm resting along your trunk.

▶ Maintain your pelvic tuck.

▶ Lift your shoulders and lower arm off the floor, allowing your top hand to slide past your hips.

▶ Breathe out as you lift, and hold the position for a moment.

▶ Release, breathing in as you lower yourself.

▶ Repeat the exercise in sets of eight. Use side-lying pelvic rocking (Exercise 18) between sets.

ADJUSTMENT

Keep your lower elbow on the floor:

▶ if this exercise is, or becomes, difficult
▶ if you have an abdominal-muscle separation
▶ as you progress through your pregnancy.

Note Do not expect to lift up very far. Your abdominal muscles will be working as soon as you begin to lift!

20
SIDE ABDOMINAL CURLS

Do both these exercises.

Starting position

▶ Lie on your side, and bend your top leg so that the knee points upwards, but keep your feet together.

▶ Support your head with one hand.

▶ Maintain your pelvic tuck through all lifts, and brace your pelvic-floor muscles.

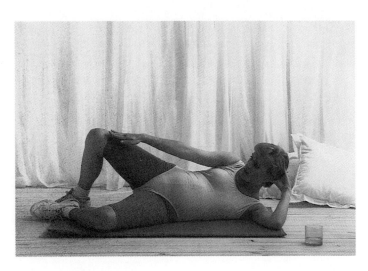

Exercise A

▶ Reach towards your top knee with your top hand, bringing your ribs towards your pelvis, and look up in line with your top knee to avoid neck strain.

▶ Release your breath as you lift.

▶ Hold the position for a moment, then lower yourself slowly to the mat.

Exercise B

▶ Reach towards your top knee with your lower hand, and look up in line with your top knee to avoid neck strain.

▶ Release your breath as you lift.

▶ Hold the position for a moment, then lower yourself slowly to the mat.

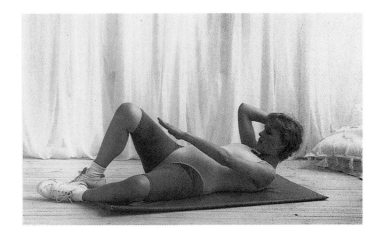

Repeat each exercise, building up to sets of eight. Use pelvic rocking (Exercise 18) as a rest between sets.

VARIATION

As your pregnancy progresses, an easier option to doing Exercises A and B is to alternate lifting your upper hand towards your upper knee (Exercise A) with lifting your lower hand towards your lower knee.

TIPS

▶ You do not have to take your hand all the way to your knee. As your pregnancy progresses, your abdominal muscles will be strengthened by holding your pelvic tuck and the attempt to raise your hand towards your knee.

▶ Brace your pelvic-floor muscles as you lift your head to prevent straining these muscles and thus reduce the risk of incontinence.

▶ To help prevent neck strain, do not pull your chin forward towards your chest as you lift.

21
THIGH STRETCHES

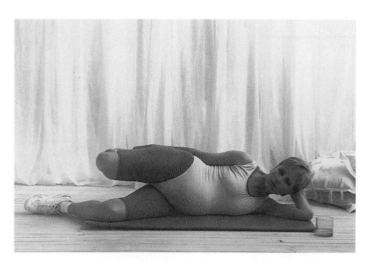

- Lie on your side, and roll forward slightly.

- Bend your lower leg forward for balance.

- Maintain your pelvic tuck throughout the stretch.

- Grasp your top ankle and gently take your knee back behind your body until you feel a stretch in your thigh.

- Keep your knee pointing forward and parallel to the floor.

- Hold the position for at least 10 seconds.

- Release, then repeat the stretch.

TIP

If you feel a stretch in your knee rather than your thigh, ease the pressure around your ankle and take your thigh further behind your body.

TRANSFERRING TO THE OTHER SIDE

‣ Lying on your side, tuck your pelvis in, then roll smoothly forward onto one hand and the opposite elbow.

‣ With your knees still together, push yourself up into a side-sitting position and then into the hands and knees position.

‣ In the hands and knees position, repeat Exercise 14 to help stabilise your pelvis. You may wish to repeat all the Exercises from 13 to 16. Then change to your other side, via the side-sitting position, and repeat Exercises 18 to 21.

Alternative method in early pregnancy

Keeping your knees together and your pelvis tucked in (to avoid strain on your abdominal muscles and pelvic joints), roll gently from your side onto your back and then to the other side.

TRANSFERRING TO THE SITTING POSITION

- Lying on your side, bring your heels close to your bottom.

- Maintain your pelvic tuck throughout the move.

- Roll forward onto your elbow and push up onto your hands (see the photograph for 'Transferring to Lying on Your Side' given earlier).

- Gently bring your feet around to the cross-legged sitting position.

CAUTION

If this position causes or aggravates pelvic-joint discomfort, you should do your upper-body exercises and stretches sitting upright on a firm chair or stool.

TIPS FOR MAINTAINING POSTURE

- Keep your legs comfortably close to your trunk.
- Sit tall, as if you were a puppet being pulled up through the crown of your head.
- Hug your baby with your abdominals.
- Take your weight evenly on both buttocks.

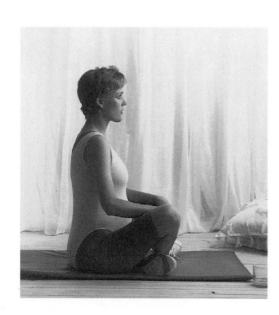

To release any tension in your back and shoulders, do backward shoulder rolls between each of the following exercises.

22

SHOULDER
STRENGTHENING 1

- Sit tall.

- 'Press-stud', or brace, your abdominal muscles.

- Brace your pelvic-floor muscles.

- Stretch both your arms up and forward in front of your face, crossing your hands over each other.

- Pull your arms down and back until your thumbs touch your lowest ribs.

- Keep your elbows tucked in and feel your shoulder blades squeezing together.

- Breathe comfortably throughout the exercise.

- Repeat in sets of eight.

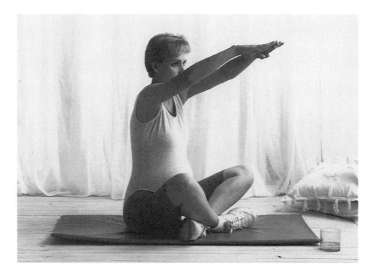

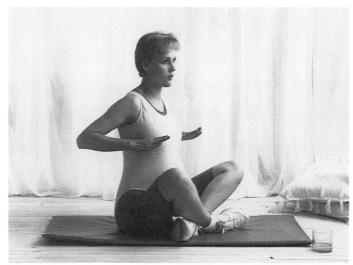

23

SHOULDER STRENGTHENING 2

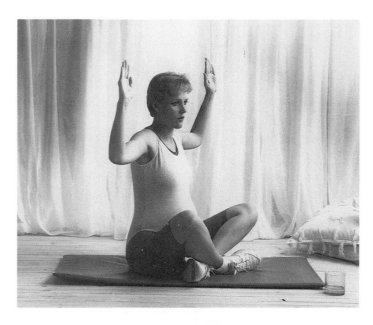

- Sit tall.

- 'Press-stud', or brace, your abdominal muscles.

- Brace your pelvic-floor muscles.

- Lift your elbows to shoulder height, with your hands up.

- Take your elbows back until you feel your shoulder blades squeezing together.

- Hold the position for a moment.

- Bring your arms forward so that both elbows and both hands come towards each other.

- Breathe comfortably throughout the exercise.

- Repeat in sets of eight.

VARIATION

To help avoid upper-back and neck tension and raising your blood pressure, you may choose to alternate sets of this exercise with sets of the first shoulder strengthening exercise (Exercise 22).

24

TRUNK STRETCHES

Do all three trunk stretches, breathing comfortably throughout.

Lift

▶ Sit tall, place one hand beside a buttock and gently push into the floor with this hand.

▶ Stretch your opposite arm vertically.

▶ Hold the position for about 10 seconds.

▶ Release.

▶ Repeat the exercise, using your other arm.

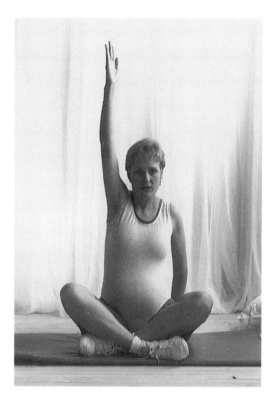

Bend

▶ Sit tall, place one hand beside a buttock and gently push into the floor with this hand.

▶ Lift your other hand.

▶ Bend to the side, keeping your trunk elongated.

▶ Hold the position for about 10 seconds.

▶ Release.

▶ Repeat the exercise, using your other arm.

TIP

The first two stretches are good for the relief of the heartburn and the pressure of the baby under your ribs that is often experienced in later pregnancy.

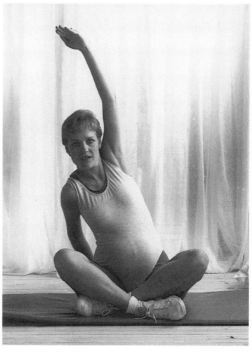

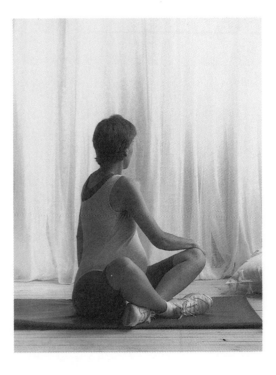

TRUNK STRETCHES *continued*

Twist

▶ Sit tall, place one hand on the floor behind your back, close to the mid-line, and gently push into the floor with this hand.

▶ Twist your trunk towards that hand.

▶ Bring your other hand to rest across your knee.

▶ Hold the position for about 10 seconds.

▶ Release.

▶ Repeat the exercise on your other side.

CAUTION

If you have a history of disc injury and any of the trunk stretches aggravates your low back pain, consult your exercise consultant for alternatives.

25

HIP AND BUTTOCK STRETCHES

- Keep your back straight and long as you sit, and look forward.

- Put your hands comfortably on the floor in front of your feet.

- Fold forward from your hips and take your weight onto your hands.

- Hold the position, when you feel a comfortable stretch behind your hips, for at least 10 seconds.

- Push up through your hands to return from the stretch.

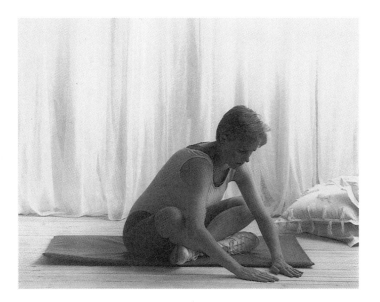

ADJUSTMENT

If you feel discomfort in your back, rather than a stretch in your buttocks, rest your elbows on your knees, then gently fold forward from your hips.

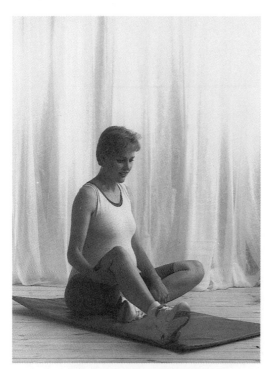

26

HAMSTRING STRETCHES

- From the sitting position take one leg out, lifting it with a hand under the knee to protect your pelvic joints.

- Sit tall, looking forward.

- Keep your elbows relaxed and gently resting on your thighs.

- Lean forward from your hips until you feel a comfortable stretch behind your thigh.

- Hold the position for at least 10 seconds.

- Release slowly.

- Repeat the stretch, using your other leg.

Note As your pregnancy progresses, your tummy may get in the way of a full hamstring stretch.

ADJUSTMENTS

If you feel any strain in your back, check that:

- your shoulders and elbows are relaxed
- your back is long and straight
- you are folding forward from your hips.

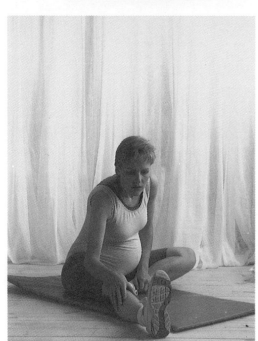

You should not be:

- twisting your back
- reaching with your hands to clasp your ankle or foot.

For a longer work-out you may like to repeat all or some of these exercises, doing them in reverse order and finishing in the standing position.

27
RELAXATION

▶ Sit cross-legged.

▶ Let your arms rest gently.

▶ Focus on your breathing and let yourself relax.

Alternative position

▶ Take off your shoes.

▶ Lie on your side with your knees bent and a small pillow between them.

▶ Rest your head on a pillow.

▶ Focus on your breathing and relax.

Note   Stay in your chosen relaxation position until you feel refreshed.

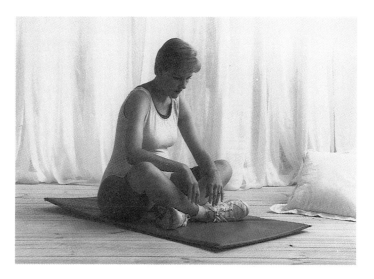

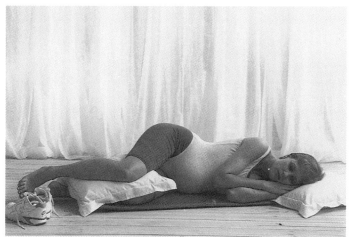

TRANSFERRING TO STANDING

From the sitting position

- Bring your knees comfortably together and to one side as you roll forward, via the side-sitting position, onto your hands and knees.

- Walk your hands back towards your feet.

- Push yourself up to a squat and then to the standing position.

From lying on your side

- Push yourself forward, via the side-sitting position, to your hands and knees.

- Walk your hands back towards your feet.

- Push yourself up to a squat and then to the standing position.

Note   Taking the time to change position in this way will help protect your tummy, back and pelvic joints from strain.

TIP

Take your time coming up into the standing position as your blood pressure may have dropped slightly. Pause a moment at each stage of your rise and tuck in your pelvis.

TO FINISH

- Repeat pelvic rocking in the standing position and then do some heel and toe raises to promote circulation. Take some deep breaths as you allow your body to squat gently.

- With your feet apart, reach your arms up to curve gracefully over your head, as you breathe in.

- Let yourself softly down into a gentle squat, with your arms curved in front of your tummy, as you release your breath.

- Repeat for a couple of breaths and finish standing tall.

- Hold your now excellent posture and walk off, refreshed.

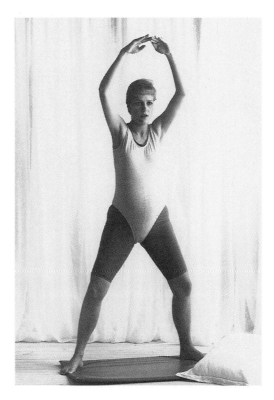

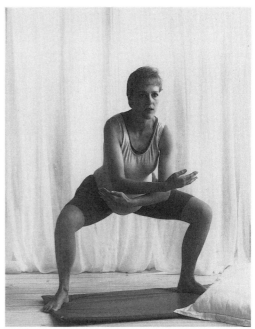

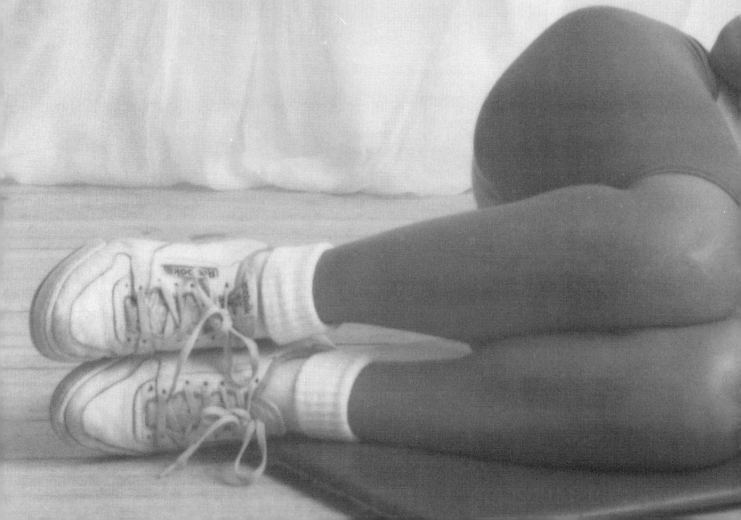

home
exercise
program
for after
childbirth

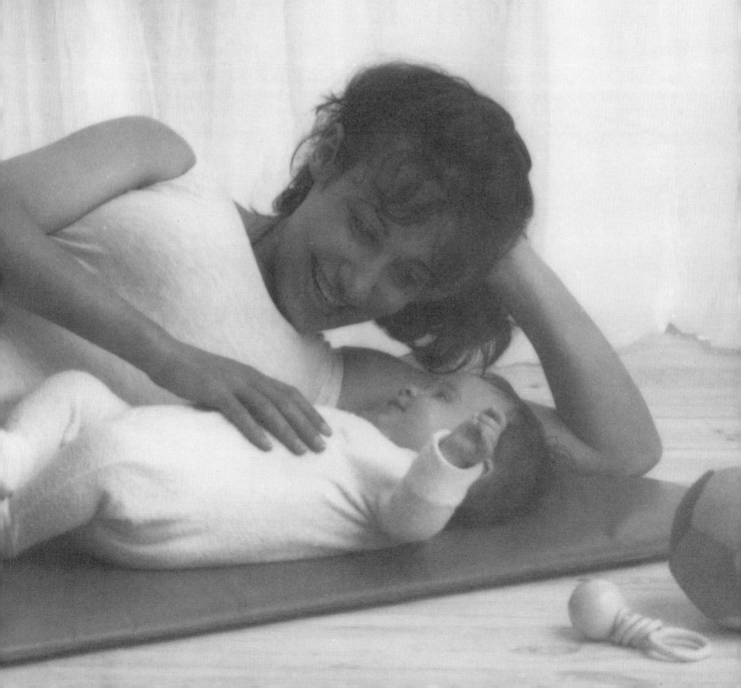

getting your body back into shape

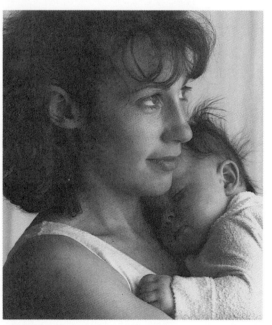

Now that your baby has arrived, you will want to start exercising to regain your shape and to increase your stamina to give you more energy in your day. You will also need to focus on postural strengthening for your new job of mothering, with all its lifting and carrying. The limits imposed by your pregnancy have been lifted, but your body is still recovering from the changes of pregnancy and the experience of childbirth and is establishing breastfeeding. So you will still need to take care with your exercise.

You may have assumed that your body would return to normal soon after your baby arrived, but in fact it takes time and work. In your rush to get back into jeans, swimwear and leotards, don't push your exercise to the limit. You may inadvertently put your body at risk of injury. Remember to be kind to yourself – give yourself a chance.

Most young mums can understand the frustration behind the common remarks: 'My clothes just don't seem to fit the way they used to!'; 'I'd love to have a little more energy left at the end of the day!'; 'I just want to tone up my body – to feel like my old self again!'. For women whose self-image is associated with their body shape, one of the hardest things to accept after childbirth is that carrying some extra fat may be a normal, if temporary, part of being a new mum. Differences in metabolism, food intake and energy expenditure mean that some women lose their pregnancy weight rapidly after childbirth, while others do not return to their previous weight until they finish breastfeeding, even though they are eating sensibly and exercising regularly.

WHEN CAN YOU START EXERCISING?

After the birth of your baby, there is a period of healing and physical adjustment. Your body is establishing breastfeeding and coping with lifestyle changes that are both psychologically and physically demanding. If you have been used to being in charge of your life, the first few weeks with a new baby can be very difficult, especially if it is your first.

During the first six to twelve weeks after your baby's birth, your body will be recovering from the effects of pregnancy and the birth. Just as an athlete understands that he or she must return to training slowly after injury, you must accept that your body needs time to repair internally and recover from the birth process, so you will also need to begin exercising gradually.

You can begin walking for exercise when you feel comfortable, and gradually increase the amount you do. Swimming should not be resumed until your blood loss (lochia) finishes, usually about four weeks after the birth. If you had a caesarean birth you may need a little longer before you feel ready to start.

It is safe to start most of the exercises in the Home Exercise Program for After Childbirth any time between two weeks (presuming your medical consultant agrees) and three to four months after your baby's birth. Your ideal starting time will depend on your birth experience and your baby's health and personality.

If you are able to commence your exercise within the first six weeks after giving birth, allow your stretched abdominal muscles to shorten, that is realign, using the pelvic rocking (Exercise 18) before adding the curl-up style of exercise (Exercise 19). If you have had a caesarean birth, you should wait until you've seen your medical consultant at six weeks before doing abdominal curl-ups or adding weights to your exercise. Ideally, whatever your situation, seek advice about which exercises you should start with from your women's health physiotherapist before you leave hospital.

WHAT CHANGES HAPPEN AFTER CHILDBIRTH?

When considering exercise after childbirth, you need to take into account a number of factors and changes that may be affecting your body.

Hormonal effects on ligaments and muscles

Your ligaments and muscles will be soft from the effects of the pregnancy hormones and stretched from your pregnant shape. Don't underestimate these as risk factors for injury as you begin exercising after childbirth. The hormone relaxin, which was responsible for softening your ligaments and muscles during pregnancy, is normally excreted from your body within the first week after the birth. However, the process of ligaments and muscles returning to their normal length and strength usually takes about twelve weeks to complete. Some ligaments around the pelvis may not return fully to their pre-pregnant state. So take care of your joints when you exercise during this time. As your muscle strength improves you will be able to do more. To protect your joints, particularly those of your back and pelvis, use:

▶ functional exercises, such as the squats and dips you will be using for lifting (Exercises 5 and 7)
▶ the pelvic tucks and abdominal bracing for postural control (see Chapter 2).

The pelvic floor

Take care of your pelvic floor in these early days of motherhood by bracing your abdominals and your pelvic floor before you lift, bend, pull, push or carry. Any exercise that builds up intra-abdominal pressure, such as resistance work, with or without weights, and breath holding while you exert pressure will cause a downward thrust on your pelvic floor. This increases the risk of a prolapse (descent) of the pelvic organs (especially the uterus and bladder). In addition, any exercise that adds impact or bounce, and abdominal curl-ups in the early weeks after childbirth, will stress the pelvic floor. Signs of pelvic-floor weakness are:

▶ a sense of heaviness in the pelvic floor
▶ incontinence (involuntary loss of urine).

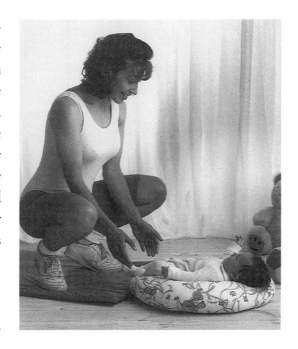

To protect your pelvic floor, be diligent about your pelvic-floor strengthening program (see Chapter 2). To help develop the holding (isometric) tone of your pelvic-floor muscles, maintain a gentle squeeze of your urethra, vagina and anus as you go about your daily activities. Continue to breathe comfortably.

To protect your back when lifting, come close to your baby and keep your abdominal muscles braced.

Abdominal muscles

After childbirth, your abdominal muscles remain stretched for quite a period. It takes time for your muscles to shorten, independent of their strength. Your urge to rush into abdominal crunches should be treated with caution! In fact, research suggests that the abdominals are not sufficiently shortened or strong enough to control the pelvis during crunches for up to eight weeks after the birth. In this period, the pelvic-tuck and abdominal-bracing exercises (see Chapter 2) and the pelvic-rocking style (Exercises 3, 4, 10, 16 and 18) are more beneficial, both for strength and posture.

As well, in these first eight weeks or so after childbirth, your lower back is not fully supported by your abdominals. It is therefore especially important to brace your abdominals when you work with your arms above your head or when you lift weights (including your baby), to protect your back. To help develop the holding tone of your abdominals, imagine you are wearing a firm corset around your tummy while you go about your daily activities. Continue to breathe comfortably.

Breastfeeding

Vigorous exercise may have an effect on your breastmilk. Your baby may not feed as well after you have exercised vigorously. As much as possible, plan your baby's feeds for before your aerobic exercise. This will also be more comfortable for you. There is conflicting evidence about whether vigorous exercise decreases milk production. The critical factor here may be the stress associated with the exercise, rather than the exercise itself. It would seem you are probably better to exercise for the pleasure of it, rather than for competition or high achievement, while you are establishing breastfeeding. Make sure you are well hydrated before, during and after exercise by drinking sufficient water, as this is another factor that affects your milk supply.

Fatigue

Allow for postnatal fatigue. When faced with the choice between rest and exercise, rest often seems to be the obvious choice. However, a balance between the two is usually best. Even though getting started may be very difficult, the good news is that mild to moderate exercise may help lessen your tiredness (depending on its cause). Exercise does make you feel good. As we have discussed, your body produces endorphins when you exercise and it's this chemical change that gives you the feeling of wellbeing. The relaxation and 'time-out' are also important benefits. So, if you're feeling a bit down or tired, try to make the effort to exercise at a mild to moderate level.

Time

You may find it difficult to make time to exercise. Babies do take a lot of care, and some babies are more demanding than others. And, as with any new job, you will take time to become proficient at mothering. You are still learning about, and adjusting to, your baby's personality and understanding his or her cries. Some strategies you can follow are:

▪ exercise with your baby, so you have a play time for your baby and an exercise time for yourself simultaneously
▪ use exercises such as pelvic tucks and abdominal bracing (see Chapter 2) to develop muscle tone and balanced posture – you can do the

standing pelvic rocking (Exercise 3) while you are changing your baby, cleaning your teeth or preparing meals

▶ set realistic goals and accept that sometimes other things, such as a sick child, may become a higher priority. Never chastise yourself, but congratulate yourself when you achieve your goals.

Use the exercises of the Home Exercise Program for After Childbirth for the first few weeks of your recovery before you return to any organised exercise, and give yourself time. With regular exercise, improvement of your awareness of your posture, and sensible eating, your shape will gradually return.

Exercise recommendations

▶ Allow time for internal healing.

▶ Begin your exercise slowly to prevent strain. Let the type and intensity of your chosen exercise reflect your stage of recovery. And remember, you should not expect to be back to your pre-pregnancy shape by any magical date.

▶ Be realistic when planning your exercise program after the birth. Allow for the physical changes that have occurred in your body — ligament laxity, muscle stretching and weakness, fatigue and breastfeeding — and the time constraints of your new job of mothering.

▶ Consider exercising with a group of other mothers so that you look forward to your work-out and time-out.

▶ Exercise to feel good, rather than to achieve competition-level fitness. Don't push yourself too hard.

FOLLOWING THE HOME EXERCISE PROGRAM

The exercise program that follows is designed for your use at home. Please note that, while the exercises are generally suitable for you after childbirth, you should consult your medical or exercise consultant for personal advice. If you intend starting these exercises before you attend the traditional six-week postnatal check-up or you have had a caesarean, make sure you take the following steps:

▶ ask your medical consultant before you leave hospital if there is anything you should be aware of that may affect your ability to exercise

▶ omit side abdominal (Exercises 17), curl-ups (Exercise 19) and advanced curl-ups with your baby (Exercise 22), until your abdominal and pelvic-floor muscles are stronger; replace them with extra pelvic rocking in the hands and knees position

▶ do the exercises the first few times with your baby on the floor nearby or while he or she is asleep, so that you can concentrate on your exercise technique.

Include in your exercise routine aerobic activities you enjoy, ideally three or four times a week, and complement them with the exercise program for strength and flexibility that follows, which has been specially designed for the early months of motherhood and beyond. The program should be done at least three times a week, but can be done daily. Like the Home Exercise Program for Pregnancy (see Chapter 6), this program is designed to flow smoothly from one position to the next, and you warm up, stabilise, work and stretch in each position before you go on to the next. For the best results you should follow the order suggested within each position. Tips, variations and cautions have been included to allow you to adjust your program to suit your body and your circumstances.

As explained in Chapter 6, the number of times you repeat an exercise is called the number of repetitions within one set. You may take a short rest then repeat the exercise set, if you wish. In the program we have often recommended that sets be made up of eight repetitions. The number of sets you do will usually increase as you become stronger. Depending on your number of repetitions, the program may last for 20 minutes.

When planning your exercise session, you should consider the following points.

▶ Allow time for these exercises. You do not have to do all the exercises every time, but don't stop abruptly. As your baby becomes more alert, make them a part of your play time together.

▶ Wear supportive footwear and loose, comfortable clothes.

▶ Exercise on a clear, non-slip floor surface to avoid accidents.

- Drink water regularly while you exercise. If it is a hot day, exercise early in the morning or in the evening, and make sure there is a good air-flow around you.
- Breathe evenly and easily during all exercises.
- To protect your joints in the early weeks after childbirth, change positions slowly and smoothly, keeping your knees together as your move.
- Never overstrain yourself: allow *no* pain. Always work within your comfort zone.
- Brace your pelvic-floor muscles during all exercises (see Chapter 2).
- Be aware of keeping a balanced posture throughout all your exercises. Always move smoothly and at a steady pace.
- Add music for your pleasure and motivation. Choose music that has a walking-pace beat. You may like to count your repetitions in eights to the beat of the music.

You can vary the program according to your needs by:

- reducing the number of repetitions you do
- choosing to do only one position each session
- repeating specific exercises
- including your baby in the session.

Now – let's get started!

the program

Each time you begin: LISTEN TO YOUR BODY.

▶ *Is it right for you today?*

▶ *Be prepared to stop exercising if you have any unusual feelings or pain.*

▶ *If any exercise doesn't feel quite right or causes discomfort (especially around your pelvis), leave it out. Substitute an easier option from the Home Exercise Program for Pregnancy given in Part 2. Try this exercise again when you're stronger or seek advice from your consultant.*

WARM-UP

Why warm up? When you begin to exercise, your warm-up will prepare your body for exercise by:

▶ increasing the blood flow to your muscles
▶ giving you a feel for movement, and therefore
▶ reducing the risk of injury to your body from exercise.

The exercises in this program are designed to flow from one to the next, so you are warming up your body as you move through the early part of the program. Adding a walk or being generally active before starting the program should ensure your body is ready for exercise.

WALKING

Go for a walk, pushing your baby in the pram or carrying him or her in a sling. Encourage your partner to join you for a family walk. Make sure you wear supportive footwear. Vary the intensity of your walk by:

▶ starting on flat, even terrain and progressing to hills
▶ varying the speed from a stroll to a vigorous walk
▶ increasing the time or distance of your walk
▶ walking with short strides and progressing to striding.

HOLDING YOUR BABY

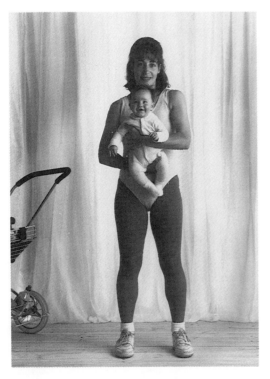

While you are doing your exercises, you might like to have your baby lying on his or her tummy to encourage him or her to lift the head. Your baby may fuss at first, but as he or she grows and wants to wriggle and roll, he or she will happily spend more time lying in this position.

If you choose to exercise with your baby in the following standing exercises, you should hold your baby in one of the two positions shown. Make sure your baby's bottom sits at or above your waist and close to your body. This will help to prevent your back from aching. These positions also encourage the development of your baby's head control.

Note If you are holding your baby, you may not be able to do sit-backs (Exercise 2), single-leg squats (Exercise 5) or dips (Exercise 7) as deeply due to his or her weight.

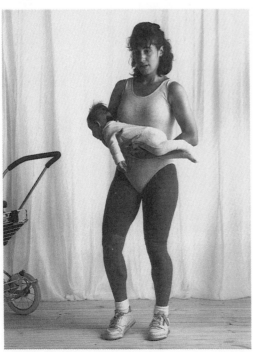

1
JOGGING ON THE SPOT

This exercise is not essential if you have just returned from a walk.

- Stand tall, with your pelvis tucked in and your abdominals braced.

- Brace your pelvic floor.

- Jog, keeping your toes on the floor, and let your arms swing freely if you are not holding your baby.

- Jog until you feel warm.

VARIATIONS

As you feel stronger, progress to the following variations.

1   March with bent elbows for extra vigour.
2   Jog as above, but punch with your fists at chest height in front of you.

2

SIT-BACKS

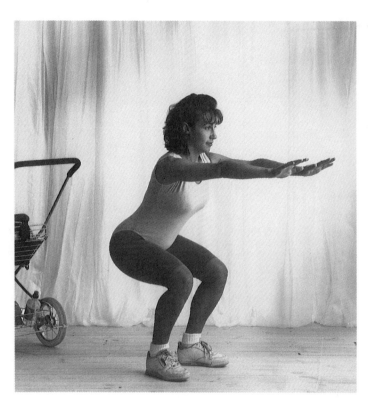

▸ Stand tall, with your feet a comfortable distance apart.

▸ Keep your weight on your heels.

▸ Sit back, as if to sit on a stool, swinging your arms forward for balance.

▸ Rise up, pushing your arms behind your body.

▸ Tuck your pelvis in to prevent your back from arching.

▸ Repeat this exercise in sets of four or eight, sitting lower as you become stronger.

▸ Between sets, jog (Exercise 1) to relieve stress on your knees.

3
PELVIC ROCKING

- Stand tall, with your legs apart and wider than your shoulders.

- Rest your hands on your hips, with your shoulders relaxed.

- Turn your toes out, with your knees in line with them.

- Bend your knees and lower your bottom to a comfortable squat position (about bar-stool height).

- Brace your pelvic-floor muscles.

- Tuck your tail under and your tummy in. 'Press-stud', or brace your abdominals. Hold the position.

- Release to the neutral position.

- Repeat in sets of eight.

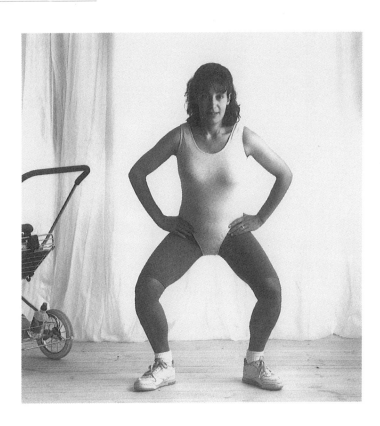

4

BELLY DANCING

Starting Position

▶ Stand tall, with your feet comfortably together and parallel.

▶ Rest your hands on your hips, with your shoulders relaxed.

▶ Let your knees bend slightly.

Option A

▶ Hitch your pelvis from side to side.

Option B

▶ Rotate your pelvis in one direction, then the reverse.

VARIATIONS

1 If you are finding this exercise difficult to do with your feet parallel, try it with them wider apart and turned out as in the pelvic rocking (Exercise 3).
2 Increase the speed and amplitude of your movements as you feel stronger, as if you were using a hula hoop.
3 Combine the pelvic movements in as many ways as you feel comfortable with (for example, side, rock, side, rock . . . *or* side, circle, side, circle . . .), or draw a figure-eight with your pelvis.

TIP

Keep the movement happening at your waist. Do not trick yourself by bending and straightening your knees.

5

SINGLE-LEG SQUATS

▶ Stand tall and gather in your waist, holding it tight.

▶ Place the toes of one foot on the ground and in front of your other foot, for balance.

▶ Rest your hands on your thighs for support.

▶ Sit back towards an imaginary stool.

▶ Repeat in sets of four or eight.

▶ Repeat the exercise, using your other leg.

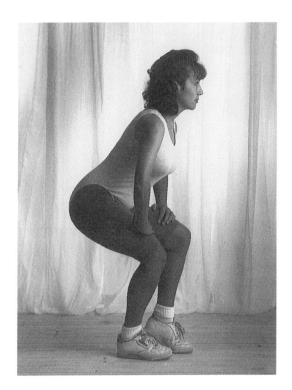

VARIATIONS

1 Lower yourself further, towards chair-seat height, as you become stronger.
2 Hold the position at your lowest position and pelvic rock before rising.

CAUTION FOR EXERCISES 5 TO 7

If Exercise 5, 6 or 7 causes discomfort around your pelvis, leave it out until you feel stronger. Substitute the squats (Exercise 7), or the chest presses (Exercise 8), or both, given in the Home Exercise for Program for Pregnancy in Part 2, to improve your thigh strength.

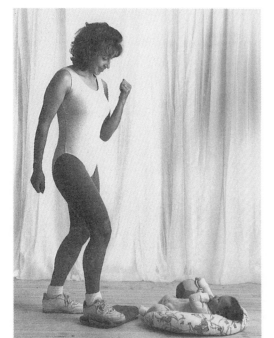

6

STEPPING

▶ Stand tall, gather in your waist and brace your pelvic floor.

▶ Let your arms swing freely.

▶ Step forward onto a marker with your *right* foot.

▶ Bring your left foot forward to join the right one.

▶ Step back with your right foot.

▶ Bring your left foot back to join the right one.

▶ Repeat the exercise, building up to a set of eight.

▶ Repeat the exercise, leading with your *left* foot.

VARIATIONS

1 Bend your elbows and pump your arms as you step forward and back, as shown in the photographs (later you may like to add a light weight).
2 Either step up onto a step or dip down as you go forward and back.

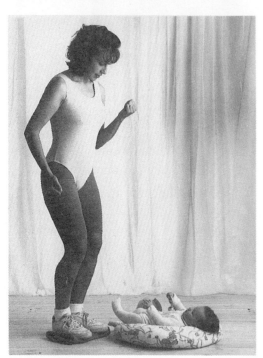

7

DIPS

- Stand tall, gather in your waist and brace your pelvic floor.

- Step back with one leg and take your weight on it.

- Maintain your pelvic tuck and keep your back straight and long.

- Lower your back knee towards the floor without lunging forward.

- Rise.

- Repeat the exercise in a set of four or eight.

- Repeat the exercise, using the other leg.

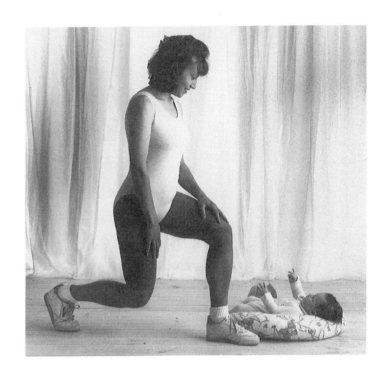

VARIATION

If your baby wants to join you, hold him or her tucked in at your waist, facing forward. Until your thigh strength improves, you may find you cannot go down as far carrying your baby's weight.

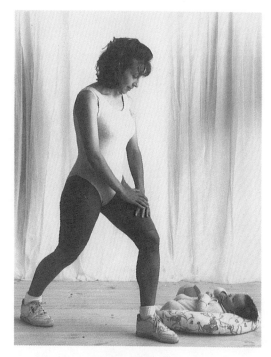

8

CALF STRETCHES

Do both these exercises.

Exercise A

▶ Stand tall.

▶ Take one leg back and shift your weight onto that leg.

▶ Place your hands on your front thigh.

▶ Press your back heel down.

▶ Look forward, keeping your back straight and long.

▶ Lunge forward, letting your front knee bend until you feel a stretch in the back calf.

▶ Hold the position for at least 10 seconds.

▶ Repeat the exercise, using your other leg.

Exercise B

▶ Take a small step in to bring your back leg towards your front leg.

▶ Take your weight on your back leg.

▶ Place your hands on your front thigh.

▶ Look forward, keeping your back straight and long.

▶ Lower your body by bending your knees, until the stretch is felt in your back calf.

▶ Hold the position for at least 10 seconds.

▶ Repeat the exercise, using your other leg.

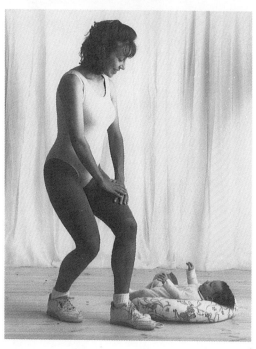

Top   Exercise A.
Bottom   Exercise B.

Use all the standing exercises as your basic work-out.
When time permits and as you feel stronger, add
some of the exercises (for example, Exercises 5 to 8)
given in the Home Exercise Program for Pregnancy in
Part 2, for a longer work-out.

TRANSFERRING TO THE FLOOR

▶ Bend both your knees and reach
down to the floor with your
hands.

▶ Take your weight on your hands
and let your knees come to the
floor.

Holding your baby

▶ Bend one knee to the floor while
hugging your baby close to you.

▶ Keeping your abdominals braced,
bend forward and lower your baby
slowly onto a bunny rug.

▶ Place your hands on either side of your baby and
bring your other knee to the floor.

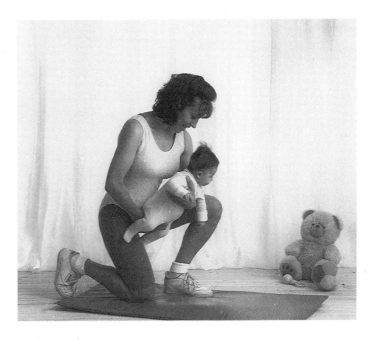

9

CAT STRETCHES

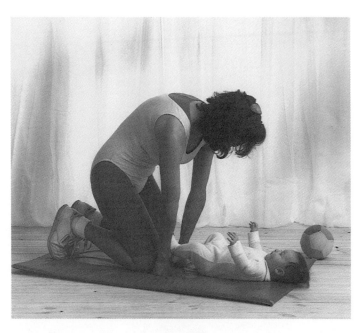

- In the hands and knees position, bring your knuckles close to your knees.

- 'Press-stud', or brace, your abdominals.

- Round your back.

- Look to the floor, tucking your tail in and your head under.

- Hold the position to feel the stretch and to strengthen your abdominals.

- Release to neutral.

- Lift your head.

- Hold the position for a moment to feel the stretch.

- Repeat the exercise in sets of eight.

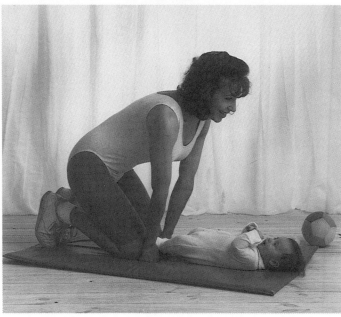

10
PELVIC ROCKING

- In the hands and knees position, take your weight evenly on your hands and knees.

- Gather in your waist and maintain this throughout the exercise.

- Round your back, and 'press-stud', or brace, your abdominals.

- Breathe out as you round your back.

- Release to neutral, breathing in as you do so.

- Repeat the exercise in sets of eight.

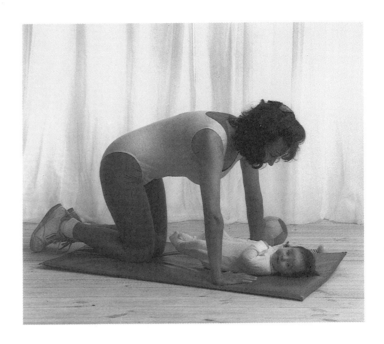

VARIATION

Take your weight on your elbows rather than your hands. This will make the rocking movement tighter.

11

PUSH-UPS OR KISSING YOUR BABY

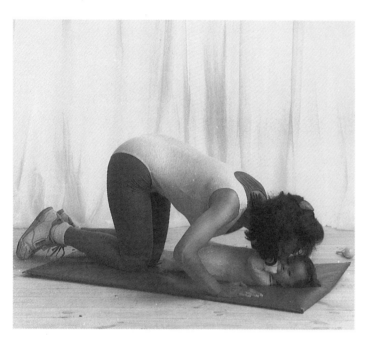

- In the hands and knees position, have your knees comfortably together.

- Place your hands on the floor in line with your shoulders.

- Maintain your pelvic tuck throughout.

- Lower yourself slowly down to the floor to kiss your baby, bending your elbows.

- Keep your back straight as you do so by holding your abdominal 'press-stud'.

- Push yourself back up, breathing out as you rise.

- Repeat the exercise in sets of eight.

VARIATIONS

1 Kiss your baby's forehead and chin alternately, to alter the weight on your arms.
2 Kiss your baby on each cheek alternately, leaning your weight on one hand more than the other.
3 Move your knees further back to increase the difficulty of the exercise (making sure your back is held straight and your abdominals are strong).

12
LEG LIFTS

- In the hands and knees position, rest on your elbows, with your forearms on the floor and your knees comfortably together.

- Lean your body weight on your forearms.

- Brace your abdominal and pelvic-floor muscles.

- Push one leg back, keeping the foot low to the floor.

- Release, and bring your knees together again.

- Repeat the exercise, alternating legs, in sets of eight.

- To realign your pelvis, pelvic rock between changing sides.

VARIATIONS

1 As you become stronger, push your leg up and out, so that it is in line with your trunk.
2 Holding your thigh horizontal, bend your knee to calf vertical position and hold for a moment. Straighten the leg, and then return to the knees together position.

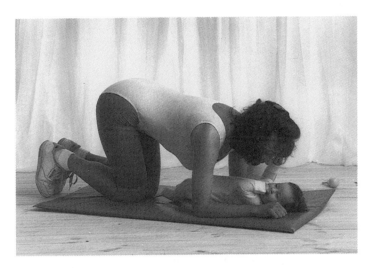

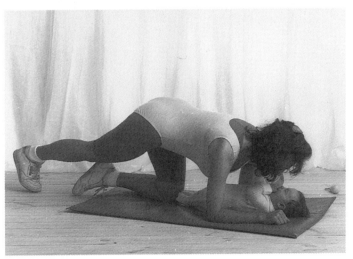

13

SIDE BENDS OR PEEP-O

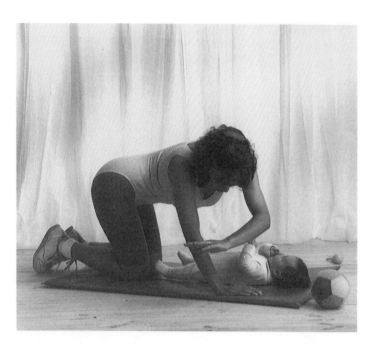

- In the hands and knees position, 'press-stud', or brace, your abdominals.

- Maintain your pelvic tuck throughout the exercise.

- Bring your right hip and shoulder towards each other, pulling your waist in as you do so.

- Swing your left arm around.

- Involve your baby by tickling his or her tummy as you pass or by squeezing a squeaky toy on one side and then the other.

- Repeat the exercise in sets of eight, reversing sides each time or doing the exercise four times on one side then the other.

14

HIP AND UPPER-BODY STRETCHES

▶ Start in the hands and knees position, with your toes together and knees apart.

▶ Sit back towards your heels until you feel a stretch in your lower back or buttocks.

▶ Hold the stretch for as long as you feel comfortable.

▶ Slide your arms forward a little to emphasise your upper-body stretch. Hold the stretch.

▶ Release, repeat the stretch and then lean forward to rest on your elbows and knees.

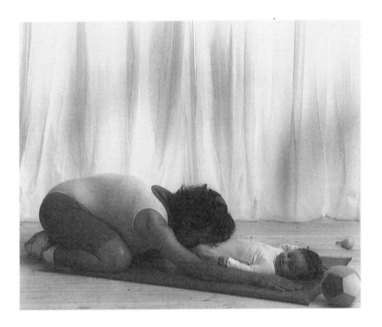

15

PELVIC-FLOOR EXERCISES

- Starting from the hands and knees position, rest on your elbows and knees.

- Squeeze and lift your pelvic-floor muscles.

- Release.

- Repeat the exercise in sets of eight.

VARIATIONS

1 'Quick flicks': squeeze and release rapidly and repeatedly, building up to about thirty times per minute.
2 Sustained holds: squeeze and hold without holding your breath, for as long as you feel comfortable. Start by holding for a count of five, and gradually build up to a count of twenty. Let the muscles relax between repetitions.

TIPS

- Keep your baby interested by:

  - talking to him or her, using different rhythms and tones for variety – your baby will soon respond with his or her own chatter!
  - change his or her position to the side or tummy.

- As well as playing with your baby, rest in this position – it's a wonderful way of relieving backache.

TRANSFERRING TO LYING ON YOUR SIDE

▶ In the hands and knees position, bring your knees together and 'press-stud', or brace, your abdominals.

▶ Gently roll your hips to one side and lower yourself, via your elbow, to the floor.

▶ If your baby is part of your exercise program, he or she will now be lying beside you.

16

SIDE-LYING PELVIC ROCKING

▶ Lying on your side, bring your knees forward and rest one knee on top of the other.

▶ 'Press-stud', or brace, your abdominals.

▶ Rock your pelvis back, as if you are pressing your back against an imaginary wall.

▶ Breathe out as you rock.

▶ Release, breathing in as you do so.

▶ Repeat the exercise in sets of eight.

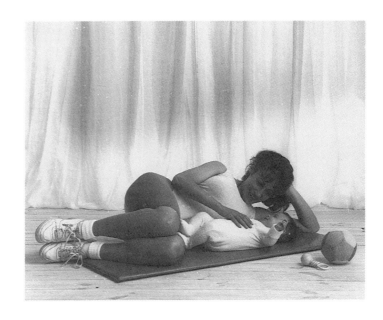

17

SIDE ABDOMINAL CURL-UPS

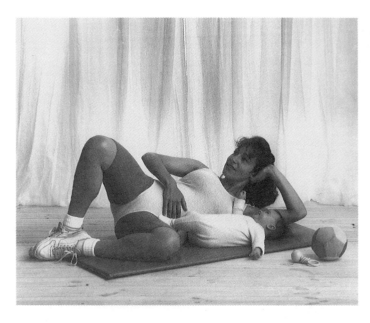

▶ Lying on your side, roll back slightly.

▶ Lift your top knee so that it points upward, but keep your lower leg resting on the floor and your feet together.

▶ Place one hand on your abdominal muscles and the other behind your head.

▶ 'Press-stud', or brace, your abdominal muscles.

▶ Brace your pelvic-floor muscles.

▶ Lift your head and shoulders, looking up to avoid neck strain.

▶ Breathe out as you lift.

▶ Release, breathing in as you lower your head and shoulders.

▶ Repeat the exercise, building up to sets of eight.

VARIATION

As you feel stronger, you may like to increase your abdominal-muscle endurance by adding the pregnancy options in this position (Exercises 19 and 20 given in the Home Exercise Program for Pregnancy in Part 2).

Repeat Exercises 16 and 17 on your other side, then roll onto your back for the following exercises.

18

PELVIC ROCKING

▶ Lie on your back, with your knees bent up and your feet flat on the floor.

▶ Lay your baby on his or her tummy between your thighs (your baby's waist should be held gently by your inner thighs).

▶ Flatten your back to the floor, tightening your buttock muscles as you do so.

▶ Hold the position for a moment.

▶ Release to neutral.

▶ Repeat the exercise in sets of eight.

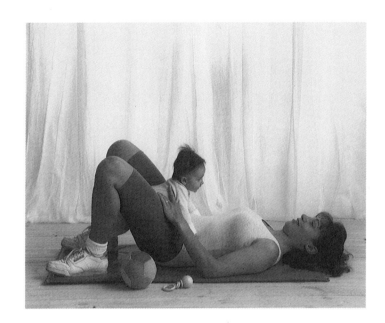

VARIATIONS

1 Lift your heels off the floor, then flatten your back.

2 Add a hold at the end of each exercise, drawing in your waist as if tightening your belt a notch!

19

CURL-UPS

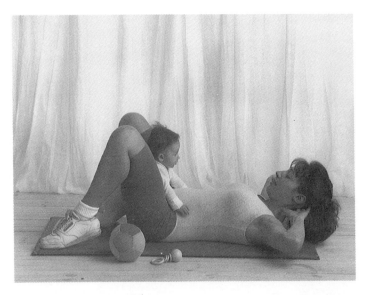

▶ Lie on your back, with your knees bent up and your feet flat on the floor.

▶ Lay your baby between your thighs.

▶ Gently place your hands behind your head.

▶ Hold your back flattened to the floor as for pelvic rocking (Exercise 18).

▶ Brace your pelvic-floor muscles.

▶ Lift your head and shoulders, bringing your ribs towards your pelvis.

▶ Breathe out as you lift.

▶ Hold the position for a moment.

▶ Release, breathing in as you lower your shoulders.

▶ Repeat the exercise, building up to sets of eight.

TIPS FOR POSTURE

▶ To prevent neck strain, rather than bring your chin to your chest, look up to the top of your knees.

▶ You do not have to place your head back on the floor each time you finish a repetition.

▶ Do not bring your elbows forward towards each other as you lift because this tends to put strain on your neck.

VARIATIONS

1 Increase the length of time you hold a curl-up.
2 Lift up a little, hold a moment, lift further, then
   hold the position. Lower your head and
   shoulders half-way, hold the position, then
   lower your shoulders to the floor.
3 Lift your head and shoulders, twist your left
   shoulder to the right, then back to centre and
   lower. Lift, twist your right shoulder to the left,
   then back to the centre and lower.

20

BRIDGING

▸ Lie on your back with your knees
  bent and your feet flat on the
  floor.

▸ Lay your baby between your thighs
  (holding him or her as shown in
  the photograph for safety).

▸ Brace your abdominal muscles.

▸ Lift your buttocks off the floor,
  squeezing your tail muscles to lift
  higher.

▸ Hold the position for a moment.

▸ To return, slowly curl your body down to the
  floor, with your upper back touching first, then
  your lower back, with your bottom last, feeling
  each vertebra touching the floor in turn.

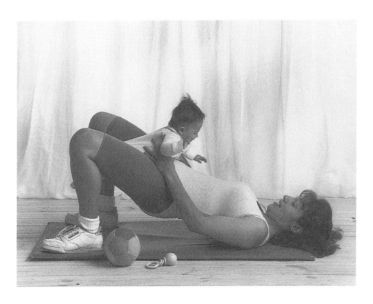

21

ROCK-A-BYE BABY

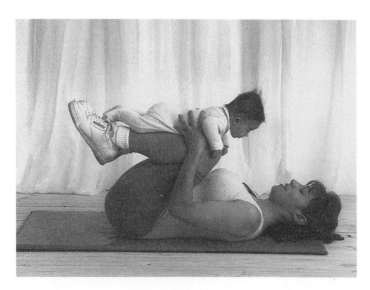

- ▶ Lie on your back with your legs bent up, as shown in the photograph.

- ▶ Place your baby along your legs, holding him or her around the chest.

- ▶ Rock your pelvis back, bring your legs towards your chest, then release.

- ▶ Repeat the movement in sets of four or eight.

CAUTIONS FOR EXERCISES 21 AND 22

1 Transferring from your back, with your feet on the floor, to this position may be difficult in the early weeks after the birth. Wait until the previous exercises are easy before doing this one. Ask someone else to place your baby on your knees and take him or her off, until you feel confident.

2 If your baby is very young, his or her head as well as body should rest on your legs.

3 Not all babies enjoy this exercise. Do not continue if your baby is not comfortable. Remember that exercise should be fun for both of you.

22
ADVANCED CURL-UPS

▶ Lie on your back, with your knees bent as in Exercise 21.

▶ Rock your back towards the floor and hold.

▶ Keep your legs still. Brace your pelvic-floor muscles, 'press-stud', or brace, your abdominals and lift your head and shoulders off the floor to look at your baby, breathing out as you do so.

▶ Hold the position for a moment, then release to the floor.

▶ Repeat the exercise building up to eight repetitions.

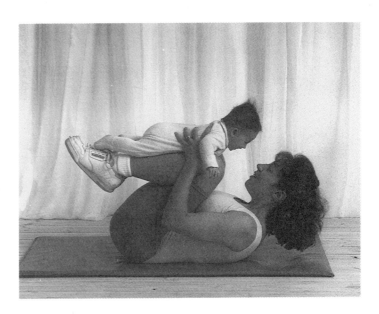

23

BACK STRETCH

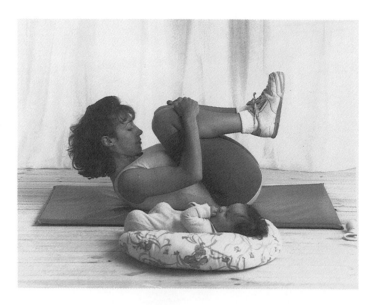

- Lie on your back, with your baby beside you, and bring your knees to your chest.

- Hug your knees firmly.

- Tuck your head under and bring your forehead towards your knees. You should not feel pressure on your pelvic floor as you lift.

- Hold the stretch for as long as it is comfortable.

- Release.

24
HAMSTRING STRETCHES

- Lie on your back, with one knee bent.

- Lift your other leg up, holding it behind the knee.

- Gently pull the leg towards you until you feel a stretch behind your thigh.

- Hold the position for at least 10 seconds.

- Release.

- Repeat the exercise, using your other leg.

Now roll over onto your tummy.

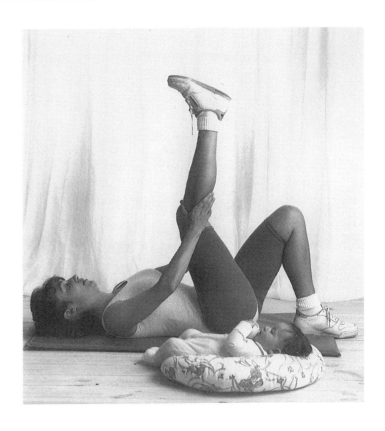

25

BACK STRENGTHENING

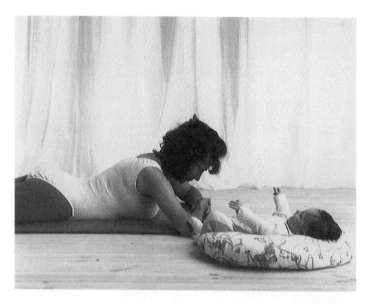

- Lie on your tummy, with your hands resting under your forehead.

- Lift your head and top of your shoulders. Keep looking at your hands so that your head remains in line with your spine.

VARIATIONS

1 Lift one arm off the floor as you lift your head, then repeat with the other arm.
2 Lift both arms off together.

CAUTIONS

- Even as you become stronger, make sure your lower abdomen and pelvis remain flat on the floor.

- If you experience any pain in your back while doing this exercise, leave it out for a while. You may wish to consult a physiotherapist for advice.

TRANSFERRING TO THE SITTING POSITION

▸ Push up from your tummy onto your hands and knees, then roll smoothly, via the side-sitting position, into the sitting position.

▸ Sit comfortably with your legs crossed.

BABY TIPS

▸ Lay your baby across your thighs, as if in a cradle, when he or she is very young (as shown in the photograph for Exercise 28).

▸ Sit your baby between your thighs with his or her bottom on the floor if he or she has developed back strength (as shown in the photograph for Exercise 26).

26

SHOULDER STRENGTHENING

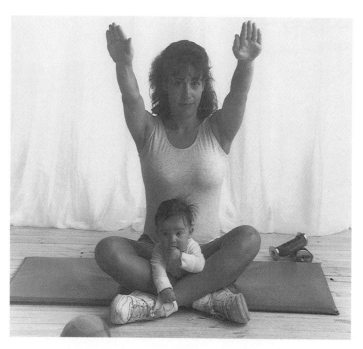

- ▶ Sit tall, with your knees gently crossed.

- ▶ Brace your abdominal and pelvic-floor muscles.

- ▶ Stretch your arms forward to about level with your forehead.

- ▶ Pull your arms down and back smoothly until your thumbs touch your lowest ribs.

- ▶ Tuck your elbows in so that you can feel your shoulder blades squeezing back.

- ▶ Repeat the exercise in sets of eight.

VARIATIONS

1 Squeeze your shoulder blades harder together and hold for a moment, to feel the opening up of the front of your chest.
2 For greater strengthening, add the second shoulder-strengthening exercise (Exercise 23) given in the Home Exercise Program for Pregnancy in Part 2.
3 Later add small hand weights to increase your strength.

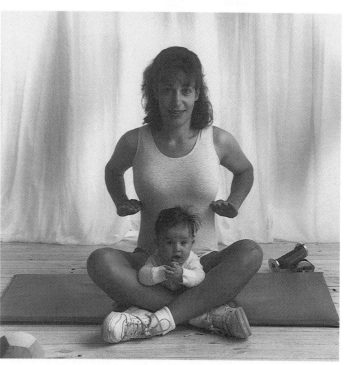

27
SHOULDER STRETCHES

- Sit tall, with your knees gently crossed.

- Brace your abdominal and pelvic-floor muscles.

- Clasp your wrists with your hands.

- Lift your arms up and back until you feel a comfortable stretch.

- Hold the position for 10 seconds.

- Release, then repeat.

VARIATION

As you become more flexible, slide your hands from your wrists towards your elbows and stretch up and back.

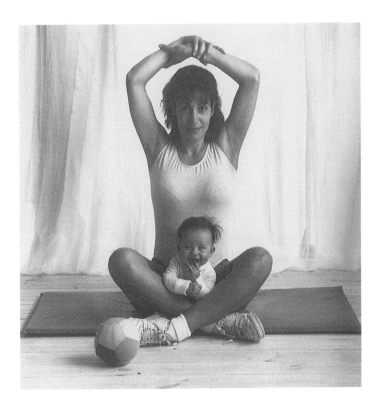

28

HEAD AND NECK MOBILITY

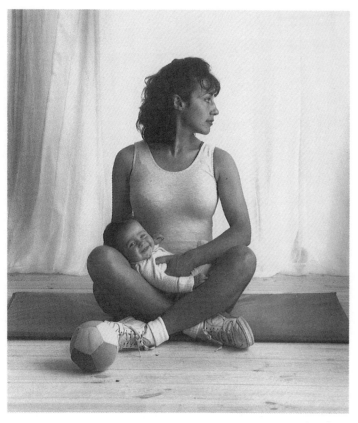

- Sit tall, with your knees gently crossed.

- Brace your abdominal and pelvic-floor muscles.

- Make sure your back and neck feel long and straight.

- Slowly turn to look over one shoulder, bring your head back to the centre, and then turn it to the other side.

VARIATIONS

1 Facing forward, slowly lower your right ear towards your right shoulder, bring your head back to the centre, and then lower your left ear towards your left shoulder.

2 Slowly let your head roll down to your chest, then roll it forward in a half-circle from ear to ear.

3 Move your head down and to one side, as if to tuck your nose under an armpit, until you feel a comfortable stretch. Hold the position. Release, and then repeat the movement on the other side.

29

HIP AND BUTTOCK STRETCH

▶ Sit tall, with your knees gently crossed.

▶ Place your hands on the floor and take your weight on them.

▶ Fold yourself forward from your hips until you feel a comfortable stretch across your buttocks.

▶ Hold the position for at least 10 seconds.

▶ Push up with your hands to release.

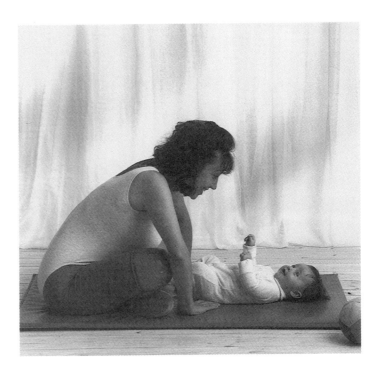

30

HAMSTRING STRETCHES

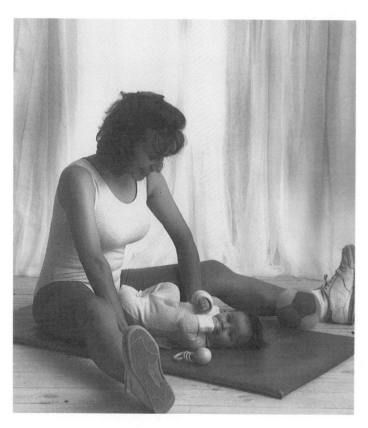

- From the cross-legged sitting position, straighten both your legs (lift them out with a hand under each knee to protect your pelvic joints if you have any pelvic discomfort).

- Sit tall, with your legs comfortably apart, and look forward.

- Place your baby between your thighs if he or she is interested.

- Place your hands on the floor on either side of your baby, keeping your elbows relaxed and bent.

- Lean forward from the hips and press your knees towards the floor until you feel a comfortable stretch behind the thighs.

- Make sure your back feels straight and long.

- Hold the position for at least 10 seconds talking to your baby while you stretch.

- Release slowly.

ADJUSTMENT

If you feel uncomfortable behind you knees or low in your back, keep your hands under your thighs and press down on your fists as you lean forward.

As your flexibility improves, this position can be a good one in which to change your baby's nappy. If you cannot maintain a straight back as you lean forward, let your knees bend slightly to avoid straining your back.

If you have time to do more stretches, do the thigh stretches (Exercise 21) and trunk stretches (Exercise 24) given in the Home Exercise Program for Pregnancy in Part 2.

31

RELAXATION

- From the sitting position, roll onto your side.

- Cradle your baby at your waist.

- Bend your knees.

- Rest your head on a pillow.

- Focus on your breathing and relax.

- Feel good about what you have done for your body, and enjoy relaxing in your baby's company.

- Rise slowly from the floor, feeling refreshed and revitalised.

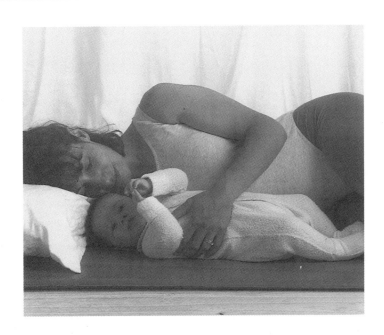

For further information about the exercises in this book or about Changing Shape classes contact:

Kathryn Bramwell
Managing Director
Changing Shape Pty Ltd
P.O. Box 256
Canterbury 3126
Victoria, Australia

Phone: 03 9888 6588
Fax: 03 9888 5433

Please note that Changing Shape is a trademarked program and registered company name (ACN 006 971160).